MIND OVER CANCER

Colin Ryder Richardson

W. Foulsham & Co. Ltd.

London ● New York ● Toronto ● Cape Town ● Sydney

W. Foulsham & Company Limited
The Publishing House
Bennetts Close, Cippenham, Berkshire SL1 5AP

ISBN 0–572–01451–1

Printed in Great Britain at St Edmundsbury Press,
Bury St Edmunds

Acknowledgements

This book is dedicated to all those whose lives are touched by cancer. May it be a stepping stone in your life's journey and inspire you to treat cancer as just another hurdle to surmount. I hope it will change your attitudes both to yourself and to those around you who love you. I trust that your awareness will grow so that you will be prepared to ask for help as you need it, know how to use the advice given for your benefit, and grow into good health as a result.

Along my journey I have been helped by many people who are all special and dear to me. They have guided me with healing hands and I offer them all my sincerest thanks. They know they have a place in my heart.

My loving thanks go to Swami Shyam who in the beginning pointed the way and continues to do so, and to my wife Rosemary who daily holds my heart and leads me out of darkness into light with tender loving care. Bless her little cotton socks.

My love to my family and friends who encourage me, help me, push and pull me upwards out of my cancerous state with great enthusiasm, and special, special love to Dottie and Greta whose healing powers enfold me, and to Sally (Crawford), my dear editoress.

Finally, to the surgeons, doctors and nurses of King Edward VII Hospital, Windsor, and Hammersmith Hospital, London. Your professional skills saved my life and gave me a chance to start my life afresh. Thank you one and all.

A note of caution

This book is written by one cancer patient to you, another cancer patient, or at least someone with experience of cancer. While the author and publishers wish to disclaim any responsibility for the methods outlined, these methods have worked for many people, including the author. But you the reader must always accept the responsibility for yourself and work in harmony with and follow the advice of your doctor.

You are unique. There will be many factors involved in your illness: your sex, age, relationships, where you live, type of cancer—and perhaps most important of all, whether you truly want to get well again at any cost.

This book perhaps will annoy you in many ways—through repetition especially, because you need, as I did, to be reminded of many truths. You may feel that I am 'talking down to you' in some way—but I assure you that this is not intended. Ask yourself instead: "Why do I feel this? Why do I react in hostility to that view? Why do I adopt this attitude? Am I being negative? Is it really me, or is it my mind making a 'monkey' out of me and somehow preventing me from getting better?".

Detach yourself from all negative thoughts and view this book in only one light: that the reason I have written it is that I want you to get yourself better. In contemplation you will learn about yourself and what you should do. Listen well to that inner voice and learn to follow what it tells you. Remember—you are the most important person in your life.

A Letter to the Purchaser

Hello,

You are probably glancing into this book to see if it is suitable for someone you know—or suitable for yourself. Possibly you have not got a cancer problem—but someone close to you has. They may be old or young, male or female, and the cancer may be anywhere in their body so the possible variations are endless. But they do all have one thing in common: they are all very, very frightened. They are all lost in life. "It happens to others', they will have said, not "to them". Good advice is needed, especially now at the start of their journey.

This book is like the first step in that journey. It is written by an ex-cancer patient. I hope it is easy to understand. I trust it offers hope to all those with cancer—and to all those who fear cancer.

If you read the letter (to the reader/patient) that begins Chapter 1, you will understand that what I am trying to do is pour my love into the very being of that reader/patient, whoever he or she is. For the very nature of cancer implies that it is the exact opposite of love.

Love is the coming together of two forces in harmony. Cancer is the chaotic splitting apart of life's energy. You must learn about the changes that take place within the body and allow the body's own healing forces to restore its natural healthy vitality.

1994.

There has been a steady demand for the second edition of this book, originally published in 1988. So will it help the reader? That is for the reader to judge. I do point out from my experience with cancer that it means a lot of effort and change on the part of the person involved, and their families—and that can be difficult.

As an example a lady in Lincoln wrote:
"Dear Colin,

I have just read your book *Mind Over Cancer* and wanted to let you know how helpful it was to me. To try to come to terms with

Lymphoma is hard and I don't like chemotherapy and all that goes with it.

I really wanted to know, are you still alive? or did it get you in the end? I hope you are well, you sound a nice, calm, gentle person and I wish you well.
Yours faithfully, R ..... H .....

In reply, I thanked her for her letter and told her that she had made my day! I confirmed I was alive and well and will remain so as long as I do not forget the "cancer lessons" which started in 1979. This book simply shares those lessons.

Sincerely,

Colin

Contents

An Invitation to Reply

This book has been written in the form of letters addressed to the purchaser, the reader (also the person with cancer), and the person who cares for them. Naturally you will not agree with all that I write but you cannot deny my sincerity in trying to help solve this problem in simple lay terms. Remember we are all unique and therefore our cancers are as varied as we are. There is no one complete answer as we each have to find our way and sing our own song. I hope I may have put you on the right route.

It has taken great inner strength to reveal what I have written. I have been propelled by forces from behind and guided through new doors that have been opened to me. There are still parts within me that are still too private to turn into mere words in a book. This I am sure you understand.

You may feel that you too have something to add and certainly I would be interested to learn your story. It could make another book! It could help others. So why not write to me in reply. All letters will be treated in confidence and I suggest that you frame your reply in the following way:—

"Dear Colin, I have recently read your book and I would like to tell you about myself and my involvement in cancer. My name is . . ." (then give your name, address, age and family circumstances);

Include a brief description of your cancer and the circumstances from which you feel it arose;

Say whether you would like further help (please enclose a stamped addressed envelope).

Send your letter to the publishers:

W. Foulsham & Co. Ltd.
The Publishing House
Bennetts Close, Cippenham, Berkshire SL1 5AP

I look forward to hearing from you and will endeavour to reply individually to each one.

Chapter 1

INTRODUCTIONS

A Letter to the Reader

Dear Friend,

If you have a cancer problem—or if you have been told that you have some sort of unusual growth—first let me say that I am sorry that you have joined the 'Big C' club. Now you have been saddled with this book to read! What a problem. You don't really want to read a book at all but perhaps you feel that you should read it. Yes, you should! So your eyes may well follow these words, but your mind will be on other things. I know, you will be saying things like:

You Why have I got cancer? Why *me*? It happens to others. It's unfair. I thought I had my life under control and now this. Look at others, they sail through life. It makes me angry. I'm frightened—and lonely. I want help—please!

Me I understand. I have been along this route. I know your feelings because I have had them.

You How can you help me? You're not even a doctor, just another cancer victim. I want proper help. I am terrified.

Me When fear reaches to this innermost part of you it is better just to shut the book, shut your eyes and breathe deeply until your heart slows down. When your mind is in a better frame start reading again.

You Sorry, Colin, but tell me a bit about yourself. If you're not a doctor, what are you? How have you cured your cancer? How can you help *me*?

Me Hold my hand and trust me. Just know that if you can open your eyes, ears and mind to all help available then much good will come. About myself: I was employed in the City of London for nearly 40 years but now work near my home as a Civil Servant. In 1979/80 cancer was discovered in my stomach. This was surgically removed and I underwent two years of chemotherapy. The chances of survival from this form of cancer are slim yet here I am, probably fitter than I have ever been, and—touching wood—I hope to be fit for a long time to come.

You Have you conquered cancer, or found a cure?

Me No. Let us just say that I am medically in remission and in that state I intend to stay. If I allow wrong influences to invade me then I am honest enough to admit that cancer will reappear within me. In that case I would be in a medical state of regression.

You I understand that after five years free of cancer you are cured.

Me The doctors might tell you that and they may be right. But I am not taking any chances. I want to stay alive, to enjoy my life and perhaps spread a bit of good in doing just that. How about you?

You Yes, Colin, I'll read your book, but I don't promise anything.

Me Don't promise me anything! Promise yourself. Don't try to convince me or anybody else, just yourself. If you find nothing in this book helpful but find a way back to good health then write *your* book.

You Once I have read your book, do you recommend other reading and if so what?

Me Yes. Read and learn as much as you can in every way. The book you hold in your hand is just the first step in your journey. At the end of this book there is a list of five Charities who can tell you of other recommended books, just search out those that you feel will give you the most suitable help.

Yours very sincerely

PS Good Luck

12

How to Read This Book

This book will contain many things that you find unimportant to you. This is inevitable when cancer is so widespread, so varied, so totally bewildering. The subject is vast, yet cancer is not a new phenomenon: it has been with us for thousands of years.

I suggest you keep a pencil handy and mark the parts that *are* important to you for ease of reference later. This is one of the things I did as I read and tried to understand what was happening to me when I learned I had stomach cancer. You could, for example, mark a section 'read again' and another 'family to read', or underline and make other suitably cryptic (or critical) notes as you go.

I also suggest that you obtain a large desk diary in which everything that is important to you is permanently recorded. Names and addresses (plus telephone numbers) of all doctors and other helpers, a careful note of all the days when you have appointments to visit the doctor, a list of the questions you want to ask and a list of the questions you have already asked and his or her answers to them. List all the things you have to do, the medicines you have to buy or that have been prescribed.

You may not wish to do this. So if you have a spouse, close friend or helper allow them to help you keep your diary. This is so important that I cannot underline enough how useful the cancer diary is to you. Even when the cancer problem is past you never know if cancer will re-occur and that diary may have useful knowledge which is not available elsewhere.

Now I did say a *large* desk diary! Hopefully you will follow my advice and record there every slightest scrap of information about yourself. Eventually you will end up knowing a lot about yourself that you never knew!

As you read on I will suggest how you can add to the diary, perhaps taking notes from this book. Eventually you will see what progress you are making. Quite often you will feel you are making no progress at all whereas the opposite will be true.

So now you have yourself in a calm frame of mind, the diary to hand, a pencil available and an unquenchable desire to conquer your problems regardless of any barriers set in your way. Read on.

Who Can Help You?

You may feel that the answer to this question is obvious: your doctor, your family, plus anybody else they recommend. These people are of course the natural choice—or are they? Your doctor may be old and his advice may need checking and updating. So do not be frightened to seek a second opinion. Be totally honest, after all you have everything to gain. Many patients treat their doctors as gods, which I suspect causes confusion (at least to the doctor), and is irksome. A doctor is more interested in a patient who has a sensible, efficient and questioning approach to their illness. Getting a second opinion can give you confirmation or otherwise of advice received. We humans are most complicated and my stomach problem was thought to be an ulcer at first but a second opinion suggested a different approach. So I am pleased that I had a second opinion otherwise I could have died just having drugs for an ulcer.

Your family you may feel are those who are closest to you both emotionally and physically and are best able to help. Perhaps in your case this could be the correct decision as it was in my case. Rosemary, my wife, gave me such strong loving support, coming with me to the doctors', seeing the doctors with me and asking the questions I was fearful of asking. She drew the line at the operating theatre but otherwise she was totally by my side. Now she tells our friends that we had cancer. Naturally this total support so lovingly given has given me the energy and motivation to fight through the years of suffering. When love is so strongly generated this strength flows through to the patient and the desire to get well again succeeds.

Look at your family. They may have their own lives to lead and having a cancer patient in addition becomes a burden they have no desire to handle. Your spouse may equally be unsuitable or unavailable and you are left to make a choice amongst your friends. The choice is yours and you must choose wisely. Your friend or helper may need to help you personally for your bodily and emotional needs. Can they handle this? Don't feel you can go it alone, even with what might be considered a lesser cancer problem. It is important to talk over all aspects and to hide nothing so your choice is important.

Usually the choice is the spouse and I will assume that like my Rosemary they will bend their lives to suit your needs, to help you in every way. Many marriages are reborn by the cancer experience provided the spouse accepts the burden from the first signs of a problem to the final signing off in the medical case notes. Alternatively many marriages finally flounder owing to the partners' inability to identify the problems which can start many years before the cancer is diagnosed. Indeed the causes of the cancer may well be rooted in such problems in early years and the cancer manifestation is the final blow.

How You Can Help Yourself

Assuming you have now selected your helper (whom I will call your spouse from now on) for the right reasons, you should take that person into your total confidence. It would be sensible if they were to read this book and help you compile your diary of useful information. Obviously you will discuss matters together and you should not hold back on any subject. You may feel you could become a bore but it is important to share your problems and thoughts so that a plan of campaign can be made. Have you considered the value of a doctor's second (or even third) opinion, for instance?

Now is the time to look up all local organisations, advice bureaux, etc who can offer you practical assistance. Your spouse can make a note of all such organisations in the diary. Your library, telephone directory, and various hospitals may all offer useful contacts that are local and so easily approachable for you. You will be offered advice, leaflets and other helpful literature and this can be gathered together and suitably noted in the diary. You may not need all of it now but it might be useful later. It is amazing just how many local organisations there are that offer help. To list all such organisations in this book would turn it into a directory and it would be out of date in any case before it was completed. Joining a local cancer group will give you a chance to compare your problems with those of others and to learn of yet further areas of help that are locally available to you.

As your diary fills up you will already start to select certain additional people from the various organisations who can help you. You will find you may like them and that they offer the kind of help you need. Your spouse can help too with enquiries so that together you are totally confident and work as a team.

Eventually you draw up your plans of what you wish to do. Remember at all stages of your treatment that you and you alone are in charge of what may or may not be done to you. You have the right to enquire, to choose and to reject at every stage. The medical area of treatment has alternatives that may be available and you must enquire. Then there are the complementary treatments as well some of which fall outside the strictly medical area. You will see how necessary it is to involve a healthy and energetic spouse to do the extra work of enquiry which you may be unable or reluctant to carry out. But even if you are in bed you can be useful with a phone so there is no real excuse for lack of action on your part. However, you will find that it is helpful to have the extra assistance.

Making the Right Decisions

What is a right decision? Some with cancer reject all advice, medication, etc and overcome their problem. Other do not and don't succeed. Making the decision that is right for you is what this book is about. It does not set out to prove that any one way is better than another. Cancer has so many forms and affects different persons in different ways. Every day medical fields open up new areas of discovery—sometimes fruitful areas leading to success, sometimes not.

Making the decision for *you* is a responsibility that is yours alone once you have all the information before you. You must be decisive and firm in your course of action. You can put your entire trust in your doctor as I did. You can help matters by positively working alongside your doctors. This is what I did as well. An attitude of "Oh, I will wait to see what the doctor says

16

next time I see him before doing anything" is wrong. Totally wrong: forget that idea. Immediate action is vital. Even if it is only in matters of diet, exercise and such like over which you are likely to have daily control.

I'm sorry to say that the one thing you cannot do is sit on your hands. In body, mind and spirit you must clear all channels for total action. If you were falling down your whole being would be involved. Well, be involved, you've got cancer!

Chapter 2

REFLECTIONS

The Past

In this chapter I would like you to reflect inwardly and deeply on yourself and your past life. The reason for this is that the cause or causes of your cancer must be found. Only you have the answers and those answers are locked within you. Your diary (see page 13) is the key to unlocking those closed doors within your mind. In order to use your diary properly, just imagine you and I are on a journey—a walk for example. I have travelled this route already and I offer you my help as a guide. When we come to difficult places we will draw closer together, even to hold hands for support when there is a danger of falling.

Hold my hand now, and trust me as we go back over your life. I will set my experience alongside yours so that you can see and compare them. In this way you may find the clues that explain your degenerative disease.

Beginning anew

Let us start with the last step in your life so far, the step you have just taken, reading the previous chapter. In that chapter I suggested that you acquire a large desk diary. What did you do mentally after reading that suggestion? Did you say to yourself "I must get a diary, this sounds a good idea"? That would have been a positive thought. Actually getting a diary and using it would be a positive act. However, you may have read my suggestion and mentally ignored or put aside my advice, feeling it could wait. Thoughts along those lines are negative and mean that you are rejecting help. Don't be negative. Throughout our journey you have to share the burden and effort of travelling. I can only guide you along in the way that I feel is best.

How to use your diary

Your objective should be to totally disgorge the contents of your overburdened and worried mind into the repository of your diary in good, sensible order. Share with it the phobias and fears of medical treatment to come, set out the options open to you in terms of treatment or no treatment. Remember that as a patient you have the final say in what is done or not done to your own body. You are in charge, and only you can agree or disagree with what is offered. These decisions require strength so naturally you will discuss them with your spouse, or the person closest to you. Once a decision is made, log it in your diary.

Recognise that the less you open out about yourself in your diary, the less is your desire to seek a permanent return to good health. Think of your doctors as garage mechanics, available to you with their expertise for limited periods only. As the owner/driver of your car (body), *you* are the person in overall charge of it. Try to complete your service manual (diary) conscientiously.

When making diary entries, it is a good idea to use different coloured inks for different types of detail. Red ink, for instance, could be used for appointments, blue ink for questions to ask your doctors, green ink for diet, black for negative thoughts and negative details about your past. As your diary with its multi-coloured inks starts to reflect your true self, you will have the feeling of peeling off many different layers, like peeling away the layers of an onion. Watch as skin after skin reveals more and more as you get towards the core. Your fears will start to surface and fresh decisions will need to be taken. Do you fight your problems, or do you run away from them? Consider your attitudes to other people. Do you always seem to come off second best? Have you been treading what seems to be the wrong path up to now?

Negative attitudes can easily build up into an endless, repeating cycle, a cycle that turns inwards into depression, despair, divorce, disease and death. The purpose of our journey then is to walk back along the pathway of your past, step by step. Could you have made better decisions? Do you regret things that you did or that were done to you? So why do you have cancer? Just know at this stage that your doctors will attend to your body's physical problems, patch you up and send you on your way. Once 'repaired', responsibility for yourself remains with 'you', not 'them'. If damage to your body was done once, it can be done twice, or more, by the same negative behaviour patterns. Reflect on this. Remember that cancer is a degenerative disease. The agency of degenerative illness comes from within ourselves.

A Record of Your Life

Re-read the first chapter and make a commitment to get that diary. Don't sit on your hands. Decide to do something new and turn afresh in a direction you may never have gone before. Reflect back on your old self, into your past, recording all the good, bad and ugly things. Day by day allow more and more things to come to the surface. Feel that you are always doing something positive, whether you are in bed or more active. Feel a surge of 'get up and go', and allow yourself to do precisely that.

Many people tell me that nothing ever happened in their lives. That in itself is a sad statement to make and could cover a whole multitude of desires unfulfilled and needs suppressed. Peel away a layer of onion skin and the record of your past will start to unfold. Peel away more skin and more is revealed, with all the joys, hurts and angers, some of which may seem trivial to others but all of which are important to you, the person concerned. It is what is important to *you* that needs to be recorded. Somehow we need to break through to the core of the stress, to the point where you can say: "can I really have hated so much and done so little?". Since I can only guide you through your past by example, I will start by showing you my own past. If and when we meet you can tell me how and why you feel your cancer was indeed the harvest of seeds of stress sown months or perhaps years before.

Finding strength in repose

I find that the mental repose gained by reflection on the past is an essential part of life. Modern life seems to be a continuous rat race leading to ever faster and more frantic lifestyles. When we are young, such hyperactivity is fun—or is it? Drink, drugs, sex and other stimulants create superabundant 'highs'. The next high has to be even higher. The next possession or experience—job, car, friend, house—has to be even more impressive. For what? Naturally I too fell for this trap. How else does one get cancer than by finding highs that have lows on the other side? I now admit the errors of my past. I cannot undo these errors but I can learn from them. As you sow so shall you reap.

In reflecting on the calm pond of my own life I see a pattern of waves that occur in roughly 10-year cycles. When I was ten years old, the second world war started. Children of my age were old enough to know fear but too young to do much about it. I was no exception. My parents lived in London and like many other families we decided to move to a safer area. A chance to evacuate to America was given to me and my parents felt that this was a sensible step. However, the liner on which I was travelling was sunk by enemy action in an Atlantic gale. Twenty hours in the sea was enough to show me the horrors of death by drowning. This experience left me shy and withdrawn, with, like many others at the time, further war experiences to endure, and I became a shy, reserved person. This was my first negative seed.

This first negative time in my life was difficult for me to handle emotionally. Boys are not supposed to cry; boys are brave and stoical. By the age of 20 I had been discharged from the Navy because of blood clots in my leg veins. My reports and the records of parade ground inspections revealed that my reserve and shyness had been clear to the naval authorities. As a result of these experiences my hair began to go white and I felt the beginnings of a stammer.

Settling down to a business life in the City and starting a family could have meant putting the past firmly behind me. But when I was 30 my father died of leukaemia. I was at his bedside with my mother and brother and afterwards we went to my mother's house to comfort her. That night my mother made her preparations and in my innocence I did nothing to question them at the time. The following morning I found that she had committed suicide in the next room. Only then did her preparations the previous night make sense. Naturally I felt this double blow most seriously. Could I, should I, have prevented what happened? Was my mother right to take her life? It was hers after all. She suffered from diabetes, but could she nevertheless have lived through the grief of my father's death? My own doubts still linger now, more than twenty-five years later.

During this time of family loss, my first wife and my children certainly did their best to comfort me. But the essential vital spark, the zest, seemed to be draining out of me. Worse than that, it all seemed to be going on without my conscious knowledge, just like an engine which loses power little by little.

By the time I was 40 I felt so drained of energy that all work became an effort. Coming home was an effort, sleeping was an effort. I tried to start new interests but I was empty within. The Church seemed no solution and I became a very confused person. Life became an endless treadmill and money seemed to get less and less. Divorce when it eventually happened, with loss of my family and the family home to my wife, seemed to be a natural conclusion to my own negativity. There seemed to be no zest in any part of my being. Talking to other cancer victims, I find their stories match my own. Sometimes their stories are worse, sometimes not quite so bad, but they all have one thing in common: they are the ones who cry and cry without tears over their past. The past represents a total bereavement so that the appearance of cancer is, if you like, the last straw in the completion of their depressing story.

Finding strength for the future

Now you must realise that my story does not end here, nor does yours. Cancer certainly appeared like the devil, suddenly taking centre stage. In my case the cancer was in my stomach, the place where I feel all hurts. The feeling I had was like the sinking feeling you get when you are about to fall. But that event was just the beginning, and through it, at the age of 50, I came to the turning point in my life.

Later on in the book you will learn how I have come to terms with my cancer with the help of doctors and many others and through my own efforts. Whether my way is your way is not for me to say. If you truly want to get well then read on. Write in the margin, marking the parts that seem important to you by under-lining in pencil or by making notes, also in the margin. Record sections that are particularly relevant to you in your diary and look to see if a pattern emerges. It will be your pattern and it will be unique to you.

Dealing with the Panic

Panic lives only in the mind. But it can be as infectious as a plague and it can sweep through a crowd (or a family), at the speed of light. Panic can shut down systems in the body as well as in the mind and it can do this either on a temporary or a permanent basis. I believe that to a greater or lesser extent we all live in such a state but that such panic is usually a negative force in our lives—that is to say it does not do too much good for our health.

When I was in hospital after my operation and was told that I had had a malignant tumour removed along with part of my stomach, the news meant nothing to me. But I could tell by the very cautious manner of approach by the surgeon, the lowering of his voice, the guarded professional manner, the screens around the bed, etc that it was obviously bad news. My second wife Rosemary and I both felt panic and burst into tears simul-taneously. Tears are an entirely normal and healthy reaction to panic. Had we tried to look bravely at one another, suppressing our grief, it would only have meant bigger problems later on. In that moment we were as one, suffering and sharing this problem equally. From that point onwards we tackled the panic problem as one—that is, together, in partnership. How many marriages can obtain that unity?

Panic, terror, fear, worry, depression, anxiety, concern and stress, are all in fact different grades of the same panic reaction. You could for example make up a scale of severity from mild upset to abject terror. None of this stress however should remain in the mind because if it does it affects the body as surely as an acid corrodes metal. The body is designed to accept a certain amount of stress in our lives otherwise we would not react properly to danger. Such a system triggers the body's emergency reaction, allowing us when necessary to run from under a falling tree or to fight off an attacker. Both mind and body are placed on full emergency and heart, lungs, muscle, eyes and so on are alerted to deal with whatever it is that has caused the reaction.

In this present age of relative peace and calm, the nervous system's emergency reaction is not normally called into play very often—until that is we introduce our own panics. This can happen all too easily in our daily lives. We can be pressed to complete a job quickly, or to handle more work and responsibility. Similarly, at home, children, telephones and housework constantly compete for attention. Stupidly, we can even seek out such stresses by watching horror films that excite us or by going for the most thrilling rides at the fun fair. All of these stimulate our nervous systems to pump out 'fight or flight' hormones like adrenalin which put our bodies into the emergency mode. Sometimes I feel we are stupid to seek out these unnecessary thrills; at other times I *know* we are!

You may well accept these views but feel that in *your* life there haven't been too many upsets. So to you I direct the following questions: do you blush easily (yes?); are you shy (yes?); are you a very caring person (yes?); do you concern yourself with other people's problems (yes?); can you easily approach a stranger and ask the way in a language you are not too familiar with (no?); can you go to your employer and persuade them to provide you with a better job (no?).

If you find that these questions and answers match your own feelings then I suggest that you are like the majority of cancer patients. I feel that these stresses can accumulate within ourselves so that they become a whole range of *suppressed stresses*. As time goes by they grow in an uncontrolled and cancerous way thus paving the way to cancer itself. As you think so shall you be.

The pathway to degenerative disease

Body stresses, whether suppressed or not, govern our attitudes and desires. The more stress is suppressed, the more the brain becomes hyperactive and the greater becomes the hyperactivity over the course of time. Eventually something has to degenerate. Hyperactivity can also be enhanced by a poor, repetitive diet especially one containing a lot of additives to which we can become unknowingly addicted.

Whatever type of person you are, you can unwittingly suppress or release enormous waves of energy, leading to a chemical imbalance in the body. I trust you can now begin to see the dangers of excessive over-activity or activity suppressed as inactivity, neither of which represents your body's normal state. Let me give you an example. When at the age of 40 I went for my motor cycle test I was in a reasonably confident state of mind. I had driven a car for many years and my motor cycle for many months. I felt confident that I would pass the test with ease. But how wrong I was! The examiner obviously disliked his job (I don't blame him). His manner was overbearing; he wielded his clipboard as if it was an automatic rifle and I was the prisoner he had in its sights. The formal requirements of the test shot out of his mouth like bullets and I could feel panic start to rise within me. The test itself was a nightmare. The engine wouldn't start, I was shouted at, the questions I was asked were impossible and the examiner's comments worse: "You have driven for 20 years without having an accident—that is unbelievable!", was a typical example. I rode home in a shaken state of mind and body. My very bowels had let me down, my confidence was zero. I couldn't believe I had actually passed. I felt somehow that I'd failed. Have you had similar experiences?

How can we become aware of the stress in our lives and the burden it does or does not place on our systems? The answer is simple. To live harmoniously, without stress, is to live in a state of joy. I like to call joy 'love' and I would like us to explore this feeling together in more detail.

Joy as a state of being does not mean drunken parties. Nor does it mean retreating to a hermitage. Being in a state of joy means carrying out your life's duties so that you gain an element of reward, of satisfaction. Call it if you like 'life satisfaction', something to look forward to with eagerness each day.

This all sounds very well, but what happens when you experience 'panic', not joy? Well firstly acknowledge this state of mind. Find a quiet place and allow your emotions to flow forth. Do not suppress the tears, do not suppress the anger. If necessary take out your rage and pain physically on some inanimate object like a pillow. You will find that a bedroom is a good place to get through this time. When the panic subsides make a factual note in your diary; eventually you will be able to see whether the periods between panics are getting longer or shorter and you will know what this means to you.

You may notice a cycle or pattern develop. With women this may be connected to their monthly menstrual cycle. Take comfort in the fact that this is a normal reaction of the brain that is felt in the body and that any suppression of the panic you feel is the last thing you should try to do. Do you find yourself saying "why me?" or "why now?"—these are classic panic statements. It will help if your spouse or closest companion does not try to smother you at these times. What you need is consolation after the panic attack is over. You will be surprised at how much better you feel. Remember that you have a natural right to express your emotions freely so long as you do not pass any of the released negativity on to someone else. Your bedroom is the best place for this private release and the relief is so rewarding. Laughter does not have exclusive rights to the discharge of your emotions.

Acceptance of Change

By now you will have noticed that certain advice on offer has been repeated; this is deliberate on my part. You need good advice and you may need that advice to be repeated many times. I hope that the advice will lead you to the same conclusion whatever your particular starting point: that is the intention. I hope that you can see an overall pattern emerging, woven like a spider's web with strands radiating from the centre and strong concentric threads to hold the whole into one. Using this pattern you can arrive at your destination by various routes. Your home of course lies at the centre and finding your very own centre is the challenge that lies within the web of your life. The story of Robert the Bruce and the spider is a well known one. The spider taught the King the lesson that whatever happens in life you do not give up. In this way you can learn to resolve your problems. You may find that you have to make changes in your life.

Finding a new resolve

How do you acquire the strength not to give up? Giving up seems so easy, even desirable, when you are at the bottom of the well of despair. However, simply crying for help when there is no-one around to hear you is not going to get you very far. So first you must accept that change is necessary. Perhaps step by step you can climb out of the well, using whatever means are available. Instead of shouting in your despair, you change tactics and accept that there may be other ways of escape.

I feel that change is essential. And that this change will mean a lot of self discovery. If you do not change, isn't your present problem likely to get worse? If you do not change, isn't your present problem likely to recur? Self discovery and improvement are the ways of change and this change can take many forms. Giving up negative things like smoking or bad diet are obvious. Less obvious but equally important is your attitude to your spouse, family, home-life, work-life, relationships and friends. Every factor in your life needs to be examined, even your reactions to reading this book. Am I, for instance, in your view, being long-winded, not getting to the point quickly enough, making you thoroughly fed up, angry or disgusted? If so, cast the book aside, don't read anymore. But you have a cancer problem; I don't any longer. Could your attitude be wrong? Look at all of these: your attitudes, your thoughts, your worries, your hopes, your loves, your future. All of them need to be examined; if any are found wanting then change is required. Think on this positively and then do what is needed. The intention of this book is to help you find your needs—you need to know what they are.

"But Colin, how can I go into hospital? Who will get my husband's cup of tea, his breakfast, his dinner?" This, seen from a woman's point of view, is an example of an inability to understand and get to grips with the need to change. The husband (it could just as easily be the wife) may be perfectly fit. But he may always have had these wifely services provided. Change is now necessary—and unfortunately this can cause resentment from the healthy members of the family. This is a dreadful problem: family routine may be so fixed that change is considered totally impossible. Nothing is totally impossible.

The Time for Action

Now! Now! Now! Now! Now! Now! So often friends with cancer say that they will wait to see what the doctor says before doing anything. Don't wait. Why wait? Cancer can act so quickly that you play straight into the hands of your enemy.

Let me tell you about a friend of mine who a few years ago collapsed with a heart condition and was taken into intensive care. With excellent medical care he survived and was advised to have a bypass operation. As he was given the choice he decided not to have the operation. Now, without it, the quality of his life is such that it takes him the best part of each morning to get up, get dressed, and have breakfast. Possibly by about 11 o'clock he is able to go for a short stroll before lunch. His whole life is like that, not much different to that of an elderly almost bedridden man. Where is the quality of life, the joy to eagerly look forward to each day? With the bypass operation he was offered, he would (admittedly with some risks attached) have been given back the freedom to live a normal life through the miracles of modern surgery. It was his choice, but did he make the right one?

I have asked this friend why he chose not to have the operation. He admits that if he had been poor and had to earn a living he would have gone ahead and had a bypass. As he is comfortably provided for he elected for a different life path. So money can be a hindrance rather than a help in getting you well. What will *you* do with the choice of actions before you? There will be no easy answer, no set solution. One person will recommend one course, someone else another. Both courses of action may give good results. The choice is yours and one you must make without delay. I understand the problems my friend had in deciding whether or not to have his heart operation: and it was a decision only he could make. My feelings, however, are with his wife who has found herself with a husband who has aged 25 years virtually overnight. My friend's non-decision (that is not to take any action), is a decision in its own right of course but he may later have to consider the consequences that arise for his future as well as that of his family. Heart disease is often degenerative in nature, just like cancer, and together they are the major killer diseases of our time. I hope that this book may prove equally helpful to those with either problem.

Making your decision well

Summoning up the courage to take any unpleasant step, perhaps in your case one where you seem to have no choice, is obviously something that needs careful thought. It might help you to make a list of the pro's and con's in your diary. Note down the possibility of taking another opinion and the various treatments you have been offered. Find out what else is available. If you or your spouse sit down with a telephone and a sense of purpose you can soon find out what help is available and bring it easily within reach. You can then make a decision based on all the available facts and feel confident that your final decision is the right one. Remember that later there will be room for further decisions; and you will make them with confidence as you learn to sift the good from the bad. If you do decide to accept a course of medical treatment you must also decide that you will see the course through to the end unless with your doctor's approval there are good reasons for stopping. The reasons do have to be good ones because your doctor simply does not have the time to debate the intricacies of your treatment at length. The more you debate once treatment starts, the less effect for good there will be. So having made up your mind, you won't change it without good reason? You will stand by your decision through all it entails? Good!

You should know that by making a firm decision, by being positive, you are actually getting better. You have kicked out all "perhaps I could have . . . maybe I should have . . ." doubts. No, you have made your decision, you are taking the right course. This inner conviction may be the first fundamental step, the most important stage in turning your life around.

Now is the time to clearly identify this positive action in large letters in your diary. Similarly record any further actions and decisions of this nature. These actions are stepping stones out of the well of despair. "If only . . . " thoughts stay behind. "I will . . . " thoughts are the way upwards out of the well. Start climbing.

Finding that 'will' to live, that zest for life, is a key to survival. If I were a really caring doctor I would instruct my medical staff to dress attractively while still retaining the appropriately professional manner of their calling; I would encourage laughter, good humour, even mild flirting—all as healthy stimuli for their patients. This kind of emotional support does happen, covertly, in many hospitals. Even matrons are known to give and receive a measure of charm that goes beyond the strict constraints of duty. To call this caring approach 'love' may sound rather excessive but that in fact is what it is—and very satisfying and natural it is too. Heart reaches to heart and gives the patient the resolve and the impulse necessary to restore the will to live. Think of the many who have been saved from death by their nurses. Such cases are often called 'miracles'. So as a cancer victim you must learn to turn the negativity of your problem into an asset. Think positive: "Here I am stuck in bed but I will see if I can get a little extra for lunch or be allowed to use the proper toilet rather than the dreaded bedpan"; "What an attractive nurse/doctor that is"; "This is certainly the good life—no work to do while others labour on having to do my work and wishing I were back". Whether you are on the patient or the healer side of the fence, open out to others with words of love, care, compassion, understanding—and do it now. Bridge the gap between you and another human being and feel the bonds that bind you heart to heart.

Strange as it may seem, if with your cancer you have started to find this new inner strength, this will to succeed, you may be the only person in the family with the ability to set out a proper plan for making the changes that are necessary. You are finding your inner strength, your will to survive is coming through. Husbands or wives will suddenly find that they are needed to do tasks they have never done before. Children suddenly need to prepare meals and get to school under their own steam. The family home may suddenly be too large for the new needs and may have to be sold.

Change may either be short-term or more permanent. Cancer brings change in many households, and as has already been said, this change is not always welcomed. Blame may come to rest on you as the cause of the change. This is obviously grossly unfair and adds a further burden. Such feelings must be discussed and dealt with in a positive manner. The best answer in such circumstances is to seek outside help. A caring outsider can view your problems in a neutral and objective manner and can suggest solutions. An experienced counsellor can offer suggestions and help that you may never have even considered. The question of what help you can expect from cancer counselling is discussed in more detail in Chapter 8.

I hope you can now accept that in taking on a counselling role, through this book, I am able to offer some of this help, that in chiding you I am chiding you lovingly, as lovingly as any parent does a child. Advice lovingly given does not always have to be taken, does not always have to be acted upon. But it does give you a chance to consider options, ideas which perhaps in your present state of mind you may have overlooked. The counsellor-parent does not function therefore as a prop, someone who gives continually, providing permanent support upon which you are dependent. The counsellor-parent relationship is one of wisdom and balance, bathed in the love of a parent, that is unconditional love. At times it will give you space so that you are free to go your own way, at other times it will hold you so closely that our hearts will fuse as one. You are as a child when confronted with cancer—we all are when confronted with any inwardly degenerative disease. So at times you will need space to act and to take that first unsupported step along your new path. "Go on, you can do it!"; there will also be the loving arms waiting to embrace you and congratulate you on your achievement.

Chapter 3

EXAMINATIONS

Your Doctor

I hope that by now you will have made some decisions about yourself following what I have written. Seeing your doctor throughout the period of diagnosis and treatment is obviously a vital point in your life, and strangely enough, many cancer patients do not appreciate just how much their lives can be affected by their doctors' decisions. The doctor's job is not an easy one and he or she may not truly understand your illness from your point of view. Your doctor may on the other hand have a brilliant hunch and decide to try some new and hopeful line of enquiry: this is obviously something you must assist in as sensibly as possible.

Have your diary to hand and rely on your spouse to give you moral support during these visits. Compile a list of important questions and make sure that you both seek satisfactory answers. It is important to ask for truthful answers and not to accept evasive ones. "How long do I have to live?"; "What are the options?"; "Will it be painful?" are direct questions and deserve direct answers. Alternatively, if you really *don't* want to know the truth, say so clearly and explain why. I don't however recommend this line of defence. What are you suppressing?

Throughout this book I concentrate on the problem of stress as being one of the main causes of cancer. Many doctors would disagree, or say that this is only partly true. Whatever the cause of your cancer, however, I can assure you that stress is one of the dominant features—not only for you as patient, but for your spouse, family, friends, business associates, even your taxman (or woman)! In other words, as your cancer spreads uncontrollably within you, its effects are mirrored in the way it affects your relationships with others. In a truly infectious way, 'cancer panic' can be transmitted to others and you should be very aware of this feature of your illness. You may not like what it does to those whom you love and trust but you must be aware of these dangers.

How to survive in the waiting room

While you are sitting in the doctor's waiting room let us look at some of the possible causes of your cancer. There may be a single contributory factor, but the causes are likely to be multiple. One of the problems with cancer is that it can take a short time or a very long time to manifest itself. You may have delayed going to your doctor thus allowing the original growth to spread. Let's look at some of the important clues: in your lifestyle, the area where you live, your diet, occupation and level of emotional stress.

Here are some possible clues to what causes cancer:

- diet—excessive intake of foods such fats, meats, sugars, salt, toxins, and food contaminants;
- smoking;
- occupational factors—asbestos, toxic chemicals, electromagnetic (X-rays) or nuclear radiation, coal dust, etc;
- sexual problems—excessive number of partners, acquired immune deficiency syndrome (AIDS), no children, late childbearing;
- emotional upsets, death or divorce in the family, depression, life dissatisfaction, etc;
- environmental factors—excessive sun, pollution, including noise and vibration, exposure to viruses.

Your cancer could arise from any of the above or from any combination of them. They can all subject your body to an abnormal and intolerable load. As your body is exposed to one abnormal stress it is more likely that other stresses will also occur. Any excess—excessive sexual intercourse, for instance— may increase worry, which may increase smoking, which may lead to depression, life dissatisfaction or death.

34

While you are waiting to see your doctor you may feel fretful or nervous, you may have a dry mouth. The first thing to do is be aware of the problem. You know that what you are about to hear may worry you. Breathing exercises will help. Shut your eyes just as if you were going to have a cat nap. Relax your body and fold your hands quietly in your lap. Breathe out, then breathe in slowly and steadily. Concentrate just on your breathing: it should be slow, deep and regular. Do not get involved in conversations with other patients; rely on your spouse to help you keep your mind rested and still for the interview. If you must talk, talk to your spouse. Allow him or her to find out the possible length of your wait; remind him or her that you need their loving help and support, that jokes in bad taste are exactly what you do not need. You are both prepared for a long wait and are pleasantly surprised when you find that before too long you are ushered in to 'the presence'.

Gaining your doctor's confidence

It is important to be totally honest once you do see the doctor. Otherwise he or she will not be able to offer you proper help. Your spouse should help you in this worrying aspect of full disclosure by being supportive. Your spouse will accompany you into the doctor's consulting room—so should your diary. You have already made a list of questions, you have brought a pen in order to record answers, and both you and your spouse should have had a final discussion to check that there are no last minute questions you wish to raise. Make sure that when you see the doctor he or she has your file open in front of them—and not that of someone else with a similar name—this does occasionally happen. You may have been asked to have a blood test a few days previously so it is useful to check whether the results are available.

Many patients feel totally overawed by their doctors. They will agree with anything and everything and afterwards they remember nothing, not even the date of their next appointment. In a word they become 'stressed' by the whole affair. And who can blame them? All doctors vary in their approach to patients. Some are unmatched in compassion *and* skill—I was lucky in this respect—while others are less good. To play your part you must have total faith in and understanding of all that is being done. Insist at the outset that you want the full truth about your condition. Say something like: "Please tell me the worst and be done with it." Get your doctor's assurance that he or she will do this and know inwardly that this will be so. And if your doctor does tell you the worst, and it proves to be less bad than you'd feared, you have the joy of relief.

In many cases, however, the doctor will be very much in the dark. With limited information coming from a terrified patient, it is amazing that any real cure ever takes place. Your spouse and your diary will back up your side of the truth, bringing out some of the things you may want to play down. You can so easily be tempted to lie about your condition. This is where your spouse should speak up, giving the doctor an honest report on your pain and suffering.

The patient's right to compassion

Doctors wear white coats, work in a clinical atmosphere, with clinical smells, and have strange bits of medical equipment about themselves. This helps provide a show of medical authority but it is in fact totally unnecessary. Doctors do not want to be confused with patients and they feed on the respect given to their office by other staff and patients alike. If this rather cruel assessment does not fit in with the impression you have of *your* doctor then you are sitting pretty.

The average doctor seems to expect nurses to produce everything they require before it is asked for. They refer to the patient as if to a machine, they dispense medication with the finesse of a magician and they seem to expect tumultuous applause as, roughly two feet above other mere mortals, they stride out of the ward. The word is 'charisma' but it is certainly not caring. If your doctor is both technically skillful, free of mistakes and also a friend to you, you are one of the lucky ones. Having watched in horror at some of the rudeness and lack of compassion that some doctors inflict on patients I feel that this is my chance for the patient to strike back. I trust you will agree that some of this anger is well justified.

The medical profession could say that I have no cause for complaint. They have provided me with a first class service and I seem to be yet another of their successes. And indeed in the vital matter of surgical skill and training I can count myself as fortunate. It is in the area of compassion and understanding, what I might call the 'bedside manner', that I feel there is room for improvement. I have listened to all the arguments on this subject and my conclusion is that in your particular case you must insist on what you feel is right for *you*. You are a human being, not a machine, and your doctor should be informed of this fact.

It sometimes helps if you comfort yourself in the presence of your doctor by indulging in the odd mind game. Start if you like by mentally stripping them of all their clothes! What would they look like completely naked? Are they overweight, do they smoke, do they drink endless cups of black coffee? Have a look at their desks for evidence of personal chaos. Do doctors answer the phone in the middle of a consultation, talk to colleagues about other matters, keep looking at their watch, make surreptitious diary notes for golfing weekends? Behaviour of this nature indicates lack of care for the patient. Such doctors are badly organised, have themselves a highly stressful lifestyle and are not good examples of self care. They themselves are on the road to cancer —possibly in your present state you should avoid such people.

Your Body

Undressing your body for your doctor to examine is a symbolic act; you are peeling off the outer layers of your physical self. First your coat, then the inner layers each drain away the self confidence you may have had when you entered the examination room. Are you ashamed of your body? Most people are, yet the body is a marvellously designed and magnificently functioning machine. Only your own mismanagement has managed to bring you to this place. You are in fact the sum total of everything that has gone before. And don't be ashamed; your doctor has seen worse! Why not feel proud of what you have? Your doctor undressed might prove to be just as embarrassed so let that thought be with you so that you could be smiling when he or she enters the examination room. As you smile try to make eye contact so that you establish a rapport, a friendship between you.

You will be questioned about any lumps and bumps or any unusual feelings within you and you must be honest in your reply. Your doctor will feel your breasts, groin, armpits and around your neck in particular; this is something you should also do when you are alone. The doctor will probe you firmly under the ribs to see how your liver is reacting and you should, if you can, try to relax. I find this difficult as I usually collapse with a fit of the giggles—but this does help to lighten the clinical atmosphere. Perhaps it makes my doctor smile and suddenly there is an infectious surge of confidence. In those moments the doctor will have reached a conclusion. The result of that conclusion could go either way: more treatment, or less treatment.

Your whole future could depend on just such a small incident as your doctor's reaction to this examination of your body. The doctor may feel that matters are getting better; there will be a belief that your body is at last responding. You identify with this confidence, and a sense of purpose and strengthening energy flows through you. Your heart beat slows down, your anxious thoughts reduce and you get dressed with a fresh hope you did not have when you first got undressed.

The doctor-patient relationship

Over-confidence is just as bad as under-confidence when it comes to understanding your body's ability to fight cancer. Your understanding of your condition must be based on absolute truth between you and your doctor. You must find that level of confidence and faith that allows you and your doctor between you to work on the problem as a team. Learn to share the decisions: "What are we going to do next?".

You may have the feeling that now that you are actually under the hands of your doctor you do not feel nearly so ill as you did before you entered the consulting room. If the doctor comes to your home, this same feeling of being slightly better occurs—"I don't know why I troubled you, doctor" is a familiar remark.

Recognise this as the confidence you have in your doctor; this causes a 'placebo' effect. A placebo is a medicine of no known action that is given to allay the patient's fears and gives the doctor time to examine the patient at a later date. Too little notice is taken of this placebo effect but it is an important one. If you feel better from whatever advice or action given or done then accept it kindly.

The Assessment Examination

The most important part of any visit to your doctor occurs after he has examined you and heard your story to bring him up to date. Have you improved? Have you stayed in the same condition? Have you got worse since the previous visit? He has the notes he has made and as he looks at these you anxiously await his reactions. If it is bad news it will be difficult for him to convey that news to you in the kindest possible way. The doctor might place the burden on your spouse before telling you. Your own feelings should be sufficiently alive to know what is possibly going to be the result of the examination. The shock of knowing you have cancer has already begun to sink in. Now, are you getting better or worse?

If the verdict is that you are getting better you leave in a cloud of happiness—you feel that it's good to be alive. Conversely, if the news is bad then you must ask all the questions which the new situation brings with it: "Will I need an operation or treatment?; What will that mean?; Can I have another opinion?; What lifespan can I expect?", and so on. If you are not able to ask these questions you must ask your spouse to speak on your behalf, the answers must be recorded in your diary so that you can consider them with care at a later time. You must decide whether you want to follow the treatment offered and if not what you intend to do. Delay is not recommended as cancer spreads so fast but once you are decided then be clear that you are not going to change your mind without good reason. Remember that *you are in control* of your body. Nobody has the right to interfere with that body in any way unless you give your permission. A firmness in your attitude to your illness must become a permanent feature of your ability to cope with it. This helps you and your doctor.

Cancer Treatments

I am not going to confuse you with the technical terms for treatments because I do not know them myself. Just because I can drive a car does not mean that I need to know exactly how the engine works—or even that it has an engine. Provided the car is properly serviced at regular intervals it should give good performance if I drive it correctly. As far as our bodies are concerned how often do we have regular check-ups? Perhaps we have our teeth checked every six months and that's about it for most people. Perhaps with regular medical check-ups we may never need the treatments outlined below.

The medical treatments you will be offered for cancer divide into three categories, variously referred to as 'cut, burn and poison':

- surgery;
- radiation therapy;
- chemotherapy.

Surgery is the oldest form of cancer treatment. The principle behind surgery is that the way to get rid of the cancer is to cut away the offending part. In many cases, in the hands of a skilled surgeon, this is completely successful. A gardener confronted with a cancerous growth on a plant would do exactly the same: cut it away to prevent any spread. Certainly as an immediate measure surgery has much to recommend it. Cutting out the cancerous tissue, however, does not mean cutting out the disease. In my view your cancer is a more complicated affair than that and the part that is surgically removed is just a symptom of something that is deeply wrong *within your self*. We will discuss this aspect in more depth as the book unfolds.

Radiation therapy involves the use of therapeutic doses of radioactive waves to kill cancerous cells. It is used particularly in lung treatment. It is ironic that radioactive material used in a controlled way can kill cancer cells and prevent them multiplying, while used in an uncontrolled way as in the atomic bombs of Hiroshima and Nagasaki, it can *cause* cancer.

Chemotherapy is the grand word used for a course of the drugs that are cytotoxic—that is they destroy cells. Since they also interfere with the processes of cell division they have been found to be effective in stopping cancer cells from multiplying.

All of the above treatments are effective but they do have severe side effects. The problems arise when the cancer has been spreading for some time before treatment is started. All the way through this book I have urged that delay is wrong—action should always be taken at once. Cancer cells can and do multiply at a rapid rate. I have learned so many times that surgeons start to operate only to discover the true extent of the disease. Sometimes in these cases it is better to close up the incision since no operation will succeed. But even a successful operation leaves problems of whether all the cancerous cells have been removed. It is also a certainty that the strength of the patient will be eroded for some time afterwards.

Having had surgery, my doctors recommended that I then have chemotherapy. Both chemotherapy and radiotherapy result in some dreadful side effects and you should enquire just how these treatments are likely to affect you. Either treatment may be given as an additional precaution after surgery and this decision depends on many factors: your age, strength and your general determination to get better. The length and strength of the treatments vary and you cannot assume that as a result of treatment you will be better or worse off than the next patient. We are all unique and just because one patient does not respond to treatment does not mean that the reaction of someone with similar problems will go the same way. This in fact is the essence of this book: you can and must find *your own* inner determination to overcome your cancer with the help of your medical treatments. I certainly found the going hard but I did not allow myself the luxury of despair or of giving up. In this I was fully supported by my wife Rosemary, and by my family and friends. Feeling weak from a major operation only to be confronted by the even bigger hurdle of two years of chemotherapy was terrifying. But it was fought through step by step. I have to say that it is your

41

attitude and the attitude of those around you to support you that will give you the necessary strength. It also requires a lot of work on your part to complement the medical treatment and we will consider this partnership in later Chapters.

How you will feel during and after treatment

Let's assume that you have fully understood what is in store for you in the way of medical treatment and see how we can overcome the possible problems in undergoing these treatments and their side effects in the easiest way possible.

Surgery: this will upset your body in every way so you need to be as fully prepared as possible. Proper mental and physical attunement comes from finding out exactly what is going to be done well in advance and physically and mentally preparing yourself for it. If you can exercise and reduce your normal workload before the operation then this is good. In my case exercise consisted of walks made up and down the ward before my operation trying to get myself as fit as possible. Take long walks, if you are able, so that you exhaust your body; this will help improve your stamina. Walks will also calm your mind because you will be able to think through the problems and realise that you can have total trust in your doctors. Going into an operation in a state of unpreparedness and uncertainty is wrong.

After surgery you will be weak. But you won't have any knowledge of what actually went on, thank goodness. Your weakness needs plenty of support from the nursing staff who will give it gladly even although they are constantly busy. The time for greatest healing is during the night, so it is quite useful to try to sleep during parts of the day as well. In this way your body is getting rest but your mind is being activated for the next stage of recovery—getting into a sitting position; getting out of bed; going to the toilet, and so on.

Night staff on wards are not always busy so they welcome the chance to talk, to support you and give you that extra care and information you need. Medical staff know that patients who are becoming frustrated by the confines of bed are getting better. I was a real nuisance, asking why I couldn't go to the toilet, why I couldn't have the tubes removed, and so on. As I asked very often so it was granted and I was able to leave the hospital within a week after major surgery. At least I gave them back their hospital bed quickly; I was going home heavily stitched up but *going home*. The first major hurdle was cleared. One final point —ever since the operation I have made it a point to take as much exercise as I can. This is to compensate for my physical loss on various levels.

Radiotherapy and chemotherapy: I have undergone chemotherapy but not radiation so obviously I know more about the former. The idea behind both treatments is to bombard the growing cancer mass that is chaotically multiplying within you. These treatments kill the cancer cells but they also kill good cells, causing possible loss of hair, softening of finger nails, etc. You may feel sick, cold, depressed, find it difficult to eat, suffer from a loss of energy and stamina and so on. These are rotten side effects and it is important to know about them in advance. You should question your doctors carefully about the likely effects these treatments will have on you. Some patients have fairly mild treatment and hardly suffer at all; others, like myself, undergo stronger doses so naturally the side effects are worse.

The positive side effects

Monitoring your treatment by making notes in your diary is important—record the days you have treatment, the length of the course, the effect it has on you and so on. You may say: "But Colin, the doctors will have all this on my file". Well yes, they will, but remember you will not always be seen by the same doctor. Your file can become quite bulky as the treatment extends over months or years. A quick check in your diary to confirm that all is correct is a sensible thing to do and will give you the feeling that you and your doctors are partners in this fight. Doctors are not almighty, they can make mistakes. You are not any less important than they are but equally important so ensure that the relationship is always on that level—a relationship of equals.

There are many types of anti-cancer therapy and all are being constantly improved. In the few years I have been involved in cancer I have seen great steps forward so my own experiences are already dated. Doctors admit that even after a year or two types of treatment change. This change is not always for the better but generally the enemy that is cancer is becoming better known. The greatest weapon against cancer is the co-operation of the patient who actually takes a positive caring attitude towards his or her own illness—for instance by reading a book like this one—and then sets out on the way that they feel is best for them. Do little and get little in return. Do a lot and find the rewards in a new and better life.

Hospitals will give you many useful ideas to support you during treatment and afterwards. You should ask for these ideas as they do make life easier for you. Here are some examples:

- Look out for a local cancer support group and get in touch. Support groups can give you so much of the advice you need.

- If you are likely to lose your hair through treatment, you may be offered a wig. Alternatively you may decide to wear a hat or a hairnet. Hair which falls out can be dangerous at night as you could inhale it, so a hairnet is very useful. I was amazed when mine fell out but as soon as it started to do so I arranged with a helpful hairdresser for my hair to be cut really short. I also sat in the sun for a short time to help reduce the difference between my white face and my even whiter skull. After a few days you come to terms with your loss of hair. When the treatment ends the hair grows back better than ever.

- Cut your nails short, being very careful not to cut the skin as the normal healing of cuts slows down. You should also be very careful about standards of cleanliness as infection is dangerous at this time.

- Avoid perfumes, deodorants, hair sprays, etc and use only plain, unscented soaps. Always ask if in doubt.

- Do not be mistaken into thinking that the treatments are having no effect. The effects can take time and you may continue to feel ill and think that your cancer has got a lot worse whereas what you are going through is actually the effect of the treatment getting to grips with the disease and causing you to *feel* worse.
- You must monitor your bowel movements and urine production carefully each time you visit the toilet. Always examine what you pass out in waste. The waste from your body is an excellent indicator of the state of your overall health. As you record your findings in your diary you may see a pattern develop. Any signs of blood in the motions, either bright red, a darker red or black, should be recorded in your diary and reported at once to your doctor. On the other hand, if the waste you produce looks good think back over the previous 24 hours and consider what it was you had to eat and drink and what activities both mental and physical you engaged in and try to repeat these over the next 24 hours. Obviously if you monitor your waste, you must also monitor your intake of food and drink, something we discuss separately.
- The effects of both radiotherapy and chemotherapy may last for some time after the particular course of treatment ends. In my own case I had two years of treatment and when it was over I felt I would forever be only half the person I was. This feeling was a depressing one but gradually the weight I had lost came back, my strength and stamina also began to improve. This improvement is very gradual and at times you will feel that you have had enough. This is when you need to find the will to carry on in the knowledge that there is a promising future ahead.
- Progress into improving treatments goes on all the time and new avenues are constantly being discovered. Always ask your doctors if in doubt. You may be offered a book or leaflet giving helpful information about your treatment and its effects. Follow this advice carefully.
- Ask about the effects on your sex life. It is likely that both sexes undergoing either radio- or chemotherapy will be told

to avoid unprotected intercourse that might lead to pregnancy.

Complementary Treatments

Many complementary treatments can be considered alongside your more orthodox medical treatments. You should first discover what is available and within easy reach. Find out the costs and anything else involved. Local cancer groups can advise you about this. Once you have completed your enquiries discuss your findings with your doctor before going ahead. I took great care in this area because although I wanted to get better I did not want to find that by taking medicines from two different sources —my doctor and a complementary therapist —I might be making myself worse. Medicines, I thought, might end up acting against one another in an antagonistic way. So whatever you feel you ought to be doing by way of complementary treatment, whether diet, exercise or anything else, first ask your doctor. Your doctor has your full medical history and it is possible that you have some other complaint as well which could prevent your getting the full or indeed any benefit.

One of the problems with complementary treatments is that there are many types offered and they are effective for certain types of cancer only; they also depend on patient and therapist maintaining the treatment on a regular basis. By that I mean that you will not get any benefit from a course of treatment that lasts say only a week. Some treatments are of the cleansing type using enemas. This can be effective in ridding the body of accumulated toxins from say the intestinal system. An example of this kind of treatment would be the Gerson Therapy. Some of my best friends offer treatments along such lines but personally I have had no such treatment as I felt that it was inappropriate for me with my particular complaint. Had my bowels been affected then my decision might have been different.

The act of cleansing the body is at the root of all good treatments. You will see that diet and the relief of stress are areas of your life which can be controlled by you and to this extent I found that I benefitted from complementary medical advice. So if you know of a local person offering a complementary form of treatment which you feel will be effective for you then go ahead with it. The actual act itself and the determination and belief in what you are doing can be just as effective as any treatment. I call this the 'will to live'.

Diet and Exercise

Most cancers are preventable. If we are only prepared to eat properly and to take plenty of exercise then we would, I am sure, not get cancers. When you do have cancer you must listen to your body and be aware of its needs rather than just stuff in what you find most attractive. If you think about it, you probably have certain favourite foods and drinks. If you constantly eat and drink these foods to the exclusion of other foods you will be depriving your body of some of its other essential needs. This leads me to another important point: if your mind is allowed to govern your body in an uncaring way it will I'm afraid allow you to stuff yourself full of total rubbish.

Diet discipline is extremely important. A diet that is good for me however may be wholly unsuitable for you. You must there-fore take good advice and be guided by what your doctors recommend. If you are undergoing radiotherapy, for instance, you should limit yourself to simple foods taken in small quantities throughout the day. It is recommended that you should avoid highly spiced and flavoured foods such as curries, onions and coffees, and restrict your diet to potatoes cooked in their jackets, fresh vegetables, fruits, eggs and soups. You should also try to drink plenty of liquids such as skimmed milk and water.

In my own case, without a proper stomach, I had to adopt a more extreme diet. I discovered the things I could and could not eat by a system of trial and error. First I had to eat little and often and I found out that the best food for me after my operation was grapes. I ate grapes by the pound all day long. I had read that a South African with cancer had attributed his cure to the eating of grapes. I found that grapes were the best thing during the first days. I then explored other foods: apples, pears, wholemeal bread, nuts, dried fruit. As my dietary choices expanded so did my physical activity. These two things go hand in hand—the more fuel you put into the body the more it needs to burn it up and so creates life energy. I also constantly monitored my bowel movements and if there was a problem I could usually discover the reason—for example putting butter on my bread meant I was having too much fat.

During the second stage, I expanded my eating to include almost all fresh vegetables and fruit, white fish (boiled), and jacket potatoes. I found I had to avoid sugar, salt, fats, including butter, meats, cheese, creamy milks, tinned foods and all fast food products. I am now in the third stage which means that I can enjoy a diet which leans heavily on the lessons learned in stages one and two but where I can sometimes mix in a bit of the items avoided during stage two. This greater dietary freedom comes from the fact that I exercise hard, getting my body to work on the food I eat. My diet has to take into account the problem of 'dumping'. This means that raw food goes straight into the gut, causing wind problems. This can obviously be difficult and is the reason I avoid highly flavoured foods. I now drink a limited amount of white wine which helps digestion.

The use of exercise to work the food through my gut has been a gradual process, building up from zero. At first I walked a few paces or climbed the stairs—and at first that was a major effort. During the time of my chemotherapy treatment I was so cold and sick that eating and exercise were the last things I wanted to do. Each day was a challenge and each day I pushed my exercise and walks further. As I got stronger, I recorded my progress across the lounge, across the street, and so on, and my diet improved. Rosemary gave me a small poodle called Honey. Now Honey needed walks and this was a challenge for me, it encouraged me to go further and further afield. Out came the bicycle so that I could give Honey a more meaningful run alongside the river. Day by day my stamina increased. I now take part in aerobic classes (run by Rosemary) on average four times a week. You must get to know your own strengths and weaknesses. You should continually ask yourself if you can do more; if you are in bed, can you sit up; if you sit up, can you get up, and so on.

Cancer can be seen as the result of the body being used badly or abused in the past. You have perhaps had upsets which have left you seriously disturbed. This disturbance of mind and body is discussed in Chapter 4. One certain way of getting rid of these problems is to work the body properly in the way it was designed to be worked. Lack of exercise is a major problem in our modern lives. Machines do all the physical work, cars save you walking, harvesters save hand reaping, there are machines that wash and clean. We are thus left with time on our hands and we get involved in more and more stressful activities without at the same time increasing our physical outlets. Seek out exercise that is good for you—walking, cycling or swimming, for instance. Ideally you should sweat out body toxins on a daily basis. So if your doctor has no objections see if you can fit in a slice of good healthy exercise to your day.

The Zest for Living

When you first learn you have cancer, any zest for living is eroded. You feel as if your life is over, that you are a burnt out cinder. Usually when I talk to others with cancer, this lack of any zest for living is often evident—*the wish not to live is being fulfilled.* The only wish is an honourable suicide. Life which has played so many dirty tricks has now delivered the final blow—cancer. Such a person shrivels in his or her shell. The idea of any zest for living is wholly rejected. I feel that this is part of the overall cancerous play. First there is depression and an increase of stress over a period of time until finally cancer manifests itself. At this stage the decline has already gone a long way and to reverse the process is like trying to save a large ship going on to the rocks by putting the engines in reverse. Whether the result will be safety or disaster depends on how soon that action is taken.

Zest for living does not consist of just one factor in your life. It has to be a whole chain of different actions which suddenly awakens you to the dangers you are running into. Depression, for instance, is a dangerous state of mind. Feeling sorry for yourself is a luxury, totally boring to everybody else. I therefore challenge cancer patients to find their own zest for living. It can be anything at all—whatever works for them. A good example in my case was getting a pet. Honey my poodle has been one link in my zest for life. There are many others of course—some, I have discovered, were already there but my negative attitudes totally overlooked them. We can all for example find a lot of things to complain about: the weather, lack of money, pressures of life, work, etc, etc. Moaning about these things upsets both ourselves and others. If they are sensible your friends will avoid you so that you will actually have even more to complain about. This will form a further stage in your physical and mental decline.

Cancer is therefore a time to challenge yourself, to challenge your attitudes, to reflect on how others see you. Just thinking about how you are may make you realise just how much of a wretch you are. So forget your negative thoughts and encapture positive things for yourself. In a way cancer is like a crucifixion, a death of an old way. Finding a zest for living, for your life, is a challenge—a challenge to find a rebirth in a new way of life, new attitudes, interests, desires, loves and wellbeing. It may involve many changes, big and small, but your life could depend on what you decide to do. Up to now you have allowed yourself to decline into a cancerous state so change *must* be the answer. This change must be of benefit to you and we will discuss this in the second part of the book. Up to now we have dealt mainly with the body. Hopefully you will have found some things which will prove helpful. I may not have given you the entire answer but I hope I may have pointed you in the right direction, to the right area of enquiry into your cancer problem.

Chapter 4

IRRITATIONS

Smoking, Drinking, Diet and Drugs

Imagine a beautiful apple, ready for picking. The sun is shining
and you know you can reach up and the fruit will release its grip
and fall from the branch. You can smell the fruit and you savour
the taste to come. Mentally you have become attuned to becoming part of that apple and the apple part of you. You hold it in
your hand, the skin breaks under the pressure of your teeth. The
juice runs down your chin as you begin to eat. Suddenly you are
aware that all is not well. The taste is not sweet but bitter. You
look at the partly eaten apple and see to your disgust that there
has been severe bruising or that an insect has been at work,
eating from the inside. You spit out the apple and your whole
desire has changed. You may select another apple with particular
care but the essence of the first desire has now gone.

Cancer is like that apple. Outwardly, in body, we appear to be
whole and desirable, but inwardly there are sinister factors at
work. An evil force is treating you like the insect in the apple.

Everyday irritants

The most everyday irritations can be an evil force if improperly
handled and understood. Supposing you are subjected to an
irritation, say excessive noise over a long period. What do you
do? Do you just accept it, or do you rebel against it? Do you find
out who is making the noise and get it stopped? Or do you go
somewhere out of the noise's range?

There are really three answers or reactions to such an irritation:

- you fight it. You find out who is making the noise and get it stopped;
- you leave it. You go out of your way to exclude the noise;
- you do nothing but suffer.

All our lives we are subjected to decisions of this nature. Each decision can be a victory, a compromise or a disaster from a health point of view and all count as possible stress points within ourselves.

Each one of us is unique so stress affects all of us differently. Some of us appear to thrive on stress, others do not. If your stresses result in victory rather than in disaster then cancer is less likely. Personal failure on the other hand encourages a cancerous pattern.

Within myself I relate very much to the idea of 'personal failure' being the cause of my cancer. Others might feel envious of my apparent successes but that fact does not help me. I just feel that they don't understand.

The pathway of irritation

To me, irritations are like standing on a cliff top. Waves are crashing on to the rocks below. The wind blows fiercely and I am aware of the danger of being perched so high up. At this moment someone pushes me hard from behind and I have a moment of pure fear as I think I am going to fall. I am sick in my stomach. It is, however, only a poor joke—some unknown person, playful at my expense, has held on to me. I have not fallen but nevertheless the stress of having *thought* I was going to fall remains active within me. If these incidents are repeated, it finally becomes difficult to truly rid oneself of such foolish fears. But consider for a moment all the mental and bodily changes they bring in their wake. The eyes widen to focus the danger on the mind, the mind activates the hormone adrenalin which flows into the bloodstream to quicken the heart and increase the breathing rate so that the muscles will have the necessary oxygen to respond quickly. Every part of the body gets ready to react instantly; the body only awaits instructions for the emergency ahead.

When we deal with such an 'emergency' by either fleeing the danger or standing to fight, we use our physical energy to work off the hormones that have put us into such a state of high alert. Then normality returns to our bodies. This is one reason why physical exercise is so important in allowing the body to work itself out of this state of high arousal.

Now consider the opposite; we set ourselves up into this highly stressful state of alert and then proceed to do nothing. *We suppress the stress.* It is not difficult to see that this must be a very wrong way of treating our bodies. Such behaviour is like revving up a cold engine, turning it off and repeating the operation again and again. Each time wastes accumulate and are not burnt off in the normal way. In our bodies these wastes tend to manifest themselves as signs of stress: nervousness, blushing, stammering, migraine, upsets in the production of stomach acid, leading to ulcers, or in my case stomach cancer.

These harmfully accumulating stress hormones can be likened to an unwanted build up of acids working within the body. As time passes, they affect the balance of the immune system. The immune system acts as the body's police force, protecting us from all villains within. But if the police force is overcome, the villains soon gain the upper hand.

External irritants

Irritations can also come from sources outside the body: smoking, drinking alcohol, eating unsuitable food, taking drugs or hormone medications such as the birth control pill. People who are under a lot of stress generally resort to smoking or drinking to relieve their pressure. They spend their time telling everyone who will listen how badly things are going for them—"look at my workload", they say. Their places of work become disorganised, so does their home, their dress, their manner. I can see some of my own friends who are following this sticky path, the same path I trod before my cancer was found. My warnings, however, are treated as if I am just trying to add to their problems rather than caring for their future. In a way such people become hyperactive, directing their energies the wrong way and eventually bringing down on their shoulders a cancer that could have been prevented.

Like many people, I know people who have smoked all their lives and have never had a day's illness. Equally I know small children who have hardly had time to do anything, certainly not anything wrong, and yet have cancer. So somewhere in each cancer patient we will find the individual problem that is unique to them. I do not have answers for all such cases, but having seen a large number of cancer victims I have been able to build up a general picture of the typical western person at risk: overfed, underexercised, worried beyond their normal tolerance. Such people get cancer.

Finding your tolerance threshold

Getting in touch with your own personal problems can be difficult. Hopefully by now we are stripping away a few of those outer layers, revealing some of your past as well as some of your present attitudes and behaviour patterns. When I was young I smoked to relieve boredom and irritations—and very good it was at doing this. Even now, after 20 years without smoking, I can still feel a desire to start smoking again. I can still feel my mouth salivate as I watch someone else in the act of lighting up and see the look of bliss at their first inhalation. Yet I loathe the effects I have seen in my friends with lung cancer, the knowledge that they have caused their cancer through their smoking—and the agony they feel that they 'cannot' give up the habit.

What do doctors do in such cases? They often feel they will create even more tension and problems if they suggest their patients 'stop smoking'. So they perhaps suggest a slight reduction. Unfortunately lung cancer is no different from other causes of cancer—it is the result of a long-term accumulation of the effects of wrong living or wrong doing.

A watch should also be kept on the consumption of alcohol, bad food, and drugs. If you are on the birth control pill, if you smoke, drink and eat a regular diet that is high in fats, meat, salt and sugar, I honestly feel that a degenerative disease like cancer is inevitable. Over-consumption of cigarettes, alcohol, bad food and drugs are all factors in the decline of your health. Ask

54

yourself: "Why did I abuse my body in such a way? What was the cause or causes?" Perhaps you were bored or it was the socially 'done thing'.

Life, Work and Play

Dealing with stress in our lives is a question of keeping it within reasonable limits so that our bodies can cope. We can all point to people who are extremely hard workers, have a lot of stress to cope with, and are at the same time very successful and happy in their lives. This is not a portrait you would recognise if you pointed at yourself. So why is there this imbalance between those whose whole lifestyle seems to create for them ever greater riches and the others? Some might say it was luck, or that they always got green lights wherever they went. Certainly looking for 'lucky' people is an art of business management. Is it just luck, or is it that the person concerned is in the right slot in their life at the right time? This is the message I try to convey to people with cancer. That they should look to see within themselves whether they are truly living as they would wish. If not, now is the time to consider a positive re-approach to their lives.

So is stress the actual bogey for your body, or is the bogey really suppressed stress—stress that is unrelieved, bottled up, allied to tensions, attitudes, beliefs, relationships lost, desires, hates, depressions, phobias, an inability to cope with life? Can these problems in their various ways manifest within you until it all finally and wretchedly comes out as cancer? Be honest; write in your diary what you know within yourself.

Your Relatives and Friends

Your spouse, your parents, your children are with you in part of your passage through life. Do you, have you, and will you truly love them with all sincerity, and will they, in return, give that same depth of love to you? You first answer: "Maybe, yes".

However, in trying to establish the cause of your cancer, no stone should be left unturned. You need to examine and re-examine what might up to now have been unthinkable to you. "Am I married to someone who truly loves me? Do my children think more of others and ignore me except for what they can get out of me? Are my parents using me? Who are my real friends?" All these questions are strong and deeply personal, but how can you live a life which on the surface is covering up a whole nest of problems below? Like snakes, these problems wriggle and menace, darting evilly whenever a crack appears.

As soon as your cancer appeared did you notice a change in the family? Did it become more united or did it somehow draw distantly apart, leaving you as an emotional prisoner, totally cold and lonely? Did the conversational tense change from: "What we are going to do", to "What we will *have* to do now"? Learn who you can trust. Let the rest run their lives their way. You need to be emotionally strong and to have a hand to guide you. At times such as this a caring outsider, such as a counsellor, can be helpful in opening your eyes to the true state of the affairs within your home and with your friends. You may realise that a form of cancer has appeared in what up to now seemed to be a happy family. Thus great strength is needed on the part of the friend or counsellor to help you through this difficult time.

"But Colin, how do I know which are which—who are the family members, friends, that I can trust?" The answer is that you look forward to seeing them with desire, enjoy their company and feel content when they have gone, looking forward to the next visit whether it is minutes, weeks or months away. That is the test. Apply it to all. Apply it to yourself as well. Would you really like to have yourself as a friend? If not, change.

Being Sorry for Your Misdeeds

If laughter is good for you, then so also should be tears. If we see someone laughing we automatically want to share the joke. Only a true friend wants to share the grief. Somehow if you feel that the points I am making are touching sore points within, that old wounds and memories are being re-awakened, then believe that they were never gone but just smouldering like a peat fire. *The anger is still within you.* These smouldering fires within the mind are awakened in dreams when the conscious suppressions are undone. Do you have bad dreams, and do they indicate that the truth within you is trying to get out?

All my life my grandfather was a model of high moral behaviour. No foul word or thought ever appeared, and yet in his last days of cancer he made up for all those lost years. I loved my grandfather, for his good and bad points, because all of that was him. It was clear to me now, however, that he was really no different from anybody else. He knew the whole range of desires and hates but he certainly suppressed them for most of this life. Was he right? Would he have been a bit more understanding in his love for his family if he had opened up? Would he have died of cancer so soon? Mind you, he did smoke the cheapest, foulest cigarettes, and he did die of lung cancer.

Are *we* as open as we should be? Do we acknowledge our sins, are we truly sorry for what we have done wrong? Do we totally repent and look for forgiveness? The idea of seeking forgiveness through repentance is, in my view, an excellent way to unburden the self of problems, provided the act is genuine and not just a chance to clear the decks for the next load of misdeeds. Carrying this load of misdeeds means carrying a cross of guilt.

Forgiveness for Your Misdeeds

Forgiveness, like love, is a two-way energy flow. Asking to be forgiven also needs the ability to truly forgive in return. Can you do that and mean it? Do you harbour anger at your spouse's misdeeds, or at those of anyone in the family or amongst your friends, colleagues or enemies? If you find there is a difficulty in doing this just acknowledge that now is not the time. Maybe the right time is around the corner. Know that the problem will continue to fester within you and when the time is right, give and receive forgiveness. Clear the slate clean of these debits. Remember it is all in your mind, nobody else's.

Learning from Your Misdeeds

My cancer is the sum total of my mistakes in life. I hope that my experiences have taught me some useful lessons. Admission of mistakes is only part of the answer though. Actually not repeating these acts of self-neglect is vital otherwise the cancer problem will recur, that is why I keep telling you over and over again why a change within you is so necessary. Others who have suffered from cancer say the same. Change *was* necessary. The quality of their lives *has* improved. Lessons have been learned and they would not go back to their old ways. How about you?

Certainly going through such an experience, with others around you suffering as well, opens your eyes. Perhaps in the past my eyes were fixed on what I did not have. I did not rest my eyes on the riches within. You must inwardly summon up the same desire to live as I did. Change that which you can and that which you want to change, and accept the unchangeable side of your life with love.

Finally in this section on irritations, you may be finding that what I write is irritating to you. If that is the case, then for you, my being irritating is a deliberate act on my part. Why? You can ask yourself why you get so easily irritated, for instance. What damage is it doing to you? Is this irritation a normal part of your being, an everyday occurrence? Does everything seem to irritate you? Yes, possibly so. Can you try to rise above this problem you have? Be honest—you may be moving towards a source of your cancer. This is important to you and needs close examination. I will try to help you if you continue to let me. Together we need to try to explore your self.

Chapter 5

EXPLORATIONS

Getting Rid of the Rubbish

We have been discussing change and I wonder if your diary is now being filled up with useful, sensible ideas of the changes that are going to occur within your future? Have you planned your next holiday? Why not? Don't give me some lame excuse. Get some travel brochures and start to instil an energy within you to get a change going. Say to your self: "I haven't time for cancer to get in the way of my life. I have much more important things to do and that I look forward to doing".

It is all a bit like spring cleaning. The weather is suddenly full of sun and energy and the home needs a fresh look. You take a look at the windows and find they need cleaning. The paintwork could do with a scrub. There are repair jobs to be done. Before you know it, you have totally cleaned up your home to your perfect satisfaction. You know it is no good putting paint on top of rotten wood, so the rotten stuff has to be replaced and then properly painted.

Spring cleaning body and mind

We are just the same in our bodies and minds. We have already considered the importance of our daily toilet waste as well as our diet—one complements the other. The exercise we give our bodies whether it is pacing up and down a ward or something more energetic, is the physical means of our beings using the food and drink and discharging the waste.

Let's examine our bodies from top to toe. It is amazing just how many people are clean in some parts of their bodies but dirty in other parts, for example their feet. You must not allow this to happen to you. We talk about washing away our sins, being purified in baptismal waters. The Bible makes many such references and so do other religious texts. There is confession, absolution and so on: these are freedoms of body and mind for which the cancer patient must have an inward desire. You may not know this yet but hopefully, somehow, somewhere in this book you will find that I have cut beneath the surface and you will begin to open out into the freedom you need.

Finding your true depths

Imagine your entire being as a pond. You can view this pond from above and from the side as if through a glass window. This is you. The surface is your skin, with various bits floating on it. Below the surface is the main body of the water. At different levels from the surface the temperature varies, so does the clarity and purity of the water. Some bits drop to the muddy floor, other bits rise like bubbles of gas. These bubbles, for example, can be your thoughts, expanding as they come to the surface, perhaps joining with others. As we grow older, the muddy floor gets thicker, the thoughts generated out of past material bubble more and more to the surface. Allowing our past to encroach on our present means that the pond is becoming more and more gassy and turbulent. The normal life of the pond changes—for the worst. The whole balance of this little world is upset into a cancerous state. Normal life disappears causing the end of the pond.

Clearing out the rubbish from your life's pond means dredging out the muck and mud from the bottom and placing it well away to create its own separate and useful compost. Your dredger is to hand in the form of your diary. Allow the past to be exposed and laid to rest as compost in your diary. Clearly, once you have done that, you will be living once more in a spring-cleaned body. Naturally there will always be some dirt on the floor and this you will need to remove on a regular basis. You will see that once you start this cleansing process the whole polluted body becomes freer of toxins, waste, corrosive acids and all the other stuff that has accumulated unwanted.

The whole concept of some cancer therapies, especially for the lower bowel, is in fact based on cleansing techniques. These treatments can be helpful if done on a regular basis so you should make some local enquiries if you feel they could be helpful to you. What you are aiming for is purity of body, mind and spirit by all the methods that are acceptable to you and your doctor, as well as being available to you locally on a regular basis.

Choices

"Colin, I am keen to get on and find a therapy that will suit me, what choices do I have?" Firstly, full marks for being keen. The spirit is there in the right place and that is so important. In fact it is possibly the most important aspect of your return to good health. Secondly, have you got rid of all those impure habits both bodily and mentally? If you were a cigarette smoker, have you stopped? If you ate a rotten diet, has that been cut out and replaced? Are the windows of your mind becoming clean and clearer? Can you begin to see the extent of the problem within you? You are not going to sit on you hands are you? Your whole attitude is one of total positive direction of energy—like my dog when she suspects that walks are about to be suggested. You might even vibrate at the thought that at last you are going to do what is required of you.

At the back of this book you will find a short list of charities who can send you a book list of further reading. Some of these books I have found helpful to me. In a few cases the titles were good but the contents disappointing. Many say the same things at various levels of understanding. All of these books were written some time ago to be in print now as I write and even as I write by the time you read *this* book many new ideas will have come forward and new books will have been written. It is up to you, with your spouse, or the person closest to you, to seek out what is most suitable for you. A book that I recommend may have helped me but may be of no particular help to you. This can cause despair so it is better for you to know the whole range of books and other information available and, in a burst of thirst for knowledge, to seek out those that contain the answer for you. I can look at many books offering excellent advice too but some are just not for me so I put them aside. Obviously the same will happen to you—but I hope not with this book.

Many people travel great distances in order to get a special form of treatment. They spend large sums in travel costs. Knowing some of the treatments involved, the question crosses my mind whether the effort involved is always worth it in terms of the treatment received. Just consider for a moment the number of people who visit shrines looking for a cure. But is it not perhaps the desire and energy involved that is part of the treatment? Is not our thirst for the present our motive for the future? A doctor will become concerned for a patient's health if they reject food. He will be happier if that same patient is asking when the next meal is coming and even happier if they can get up and get what they want themselves.

I am going therefore to offer as a 'carrot' the fact that there are many ways to get better, that the choices are all around you, that you are not the only ill person—many are much worse than you are and have found their way through. So go to it. Remember the story of the king who was ill and was prescribed a beaker of early morning dew by his doctor. After a week, the king was worse, and the doctor asked him who gathered the dew every morning—"naturally my servants", the king replied. "That is not the treatment", said the doctor, "You must personally gather the beakerful of dew and drink it".

What is Available to You

As I said, you would be amazed at the number of different things that are available to help you. Listed at the back of the book are some of the organisations that can offer this help. If they cannot themselves provide what is required they will probably be able to put you in touch with someone who can and it may be that they are just around the corner from where you live. Cancer can be seen as the disease that induces the greatest fear in the largest number of the population—young and old—so there has been a spontaneous growth of cancer organisations springing up everywhere and dedicated to assisting you.

Those who have had cancer and are prepared to get involved in this work find that they soon draw in a number of similarly inspired people nearby. The energy generated by this work soon reaches the newspapers, the local advice bureaux, local authorities, hospitals, hospices, the Samaritans, and many others. There is a wealth of experience and assistance within your reach. All you have to do is have the courage to make the contact and the dedication to your self-interest to listen to the advice given. Just reach out.

I realise that part of the whole cancer experience is to want to just throw in the towel. The "What's the use, I really want to die" attitude. It is that attitude of negativity that you must confront head-on. I can offer you the best treatments in the world but if you, that part deep inside you, will not respond and will not summon up the inclination, then it is of no use. Finding the inclination—the physical and mental slope up which you climb to good health—is what this book is all about. It is a message that I myself have to remember time and time again. Negative thinking is an easy luxury. Self-pity is a cancerous attitude. So get rid of the rubbish. What is available starts with *you*, now.

How Committed are You?

Much of our commitment to finding good health is tempered with "Oh yes, but . . ." Again this is negative thinking. Mothers tell me that their children come first. That seems so beautiful and natural. Of course children are entitled to a priority. But how high is that priority? Supposing you have to go into hospital for treatment and the children are left in the care of others. Are you going to cut short your treatment or even refuse to have it for the sake of the children? Cancer patients lose sight of their priorities in the face of fear. Good advice is ignored, and frankly foolish actions make matters many times worse.

At times like these you must recognise that you cannot always be on hand to fulfil your normal duties. There is a time to let go of such matters and to pass them into other hands and this is the time. Amazingly, life can go on without you. Your attitude to committing yourself totally to your own wellbeing is now paramount. This is a 100 per cent priority and you must understand this; others must continue their lives without your assistance and all your energies must be directed towards your own wellbeing.

Using Your Family and Friends

Once you commit yourself totally to your goal of self improvement and good health, why not use the energy of others for your benefit? Family and friends can do one of two things. Negatively, they can recoil in horror at your news and not wish to be involved at any level. Even a shoulder to cry on is given sparingly and with embarrassment. You should be prepared for this and act accordingly. I find that in such families, members create an invisible barrier to the outside world. The cancer patient is terribly alone within a kind of prison. Only nurses and doctors cross the lonely divide. Cancer helpers are told that the patient is 'too ill', or 'resting', or some other excuse is offered like 'let's wait and see'. My heart goes out to the patient who is desperately in need of loving comfort and care. All too often I find that I end up listening to the lesser problems of the rest of the family. The cancer patient's problems are set aside. In such circumstances, you, as the patient, must fight your way out of such a situation if it does develop. You could be left on your own, isolated from all help and that is certainly not as it should be. So fight through these barriers.

In a similar way, you could find that your 'friends' visit you just to find out how much worse you are, and to tell you how quickly cancer has spread in someone else they know. They eat your grapes and leave you before you have a chance to ask them if they can help you. Probably you feel you don't really want to see such people because they upset you. Perhaps they start smoking in front of you and talk about the horrors of lung cancer. Probably they will wring their hands.

My advice is don't have them around at all, whoever they are. The test is if you feel worse after a visit—then, regardless of who they are, make sure they do not visit you again. The rule is either they don't see you or you find a way of getting yourself into a more caring environment.

Family and friends can also of course bring a positive attitude. Such family and friends will visit you regardless of their own duties and commitments. They will stay as long or as short a time as you need them and they will bring a vital energy into your being and assist you in every way they can. In a way you need to sucker on to the love they bring into your world. Be certain that they know just what their love means to you. Do not be embarrassed to ask for help—just ask. Learn to receive.

The special needs of children

When there is cancer in the family, children must be told the truth. They can give their love and energy as you need it, and when you cannot handle it they should be gently told to go elsewhere so that you can get the rest you need. Your needs are absolutely vital and your assessment of your family and friends and their relationship to you is a most important factor in your wellbeing. You cannot avoid being emotionally upset; what you must decide is who within your circle of family and friends can give you the best support, the support that you need.

Finding the Right Course

There is always more than one way of solving the problems that confront a cancer patient. Making the right choice for the course of action that is best for you can be difficult. We have already considered the question of selecting within your family and friends those who can best help you. If you feel better, strengthened by a person's presence then that feeling must be encouraged. If you do not look forward to meeting even a close member of the family—say your mother—then do not allow those meetings to occur. Some family relationships can totally drain you. If that is the case then don't let it happen.

In exactly the same way you need to decide the course of action that is right for you. I am not going to suggest that you should do one thing rather than another—that is for you to decide. You have time to reflect and to consider and once you are certain that you are going for example to have treatment, to change your job, or to change whatever it is that is causing stress in your life, then make up your mind and do it. This is not a time for half measures, nor for constantly wavering between doing and not doing. Looking for excuses to cover up lack of decision is wrong.

What you are looking for are what I call 'executive' decisions. Here are some examples:

- You decide that your relationship with a particular person is draining. You then politely but firmly make sure that that person is no longer involved in your fight;
- You decide that you will take treatment;
- You decide that your diet needs revision, that you are not going to simply conform to the dietary choices in your family if that doesn't suit you;
- You decide you will eat regular small meals instead of a few big meals;
- You decide you will take more exercise;
- You decide that negative, depressing talk about the weather, money problems, emotional relationships, other people's problems are not for you;
- You decide that you are going to plan a fresh life, a new future where you will take centre stage rather than being shoved emotionally into the wings;
- You will look for the good in yourself and others. You will kick out all feelings such as that you have no place in your home, or in your job, or in the world — of course you have.

Your space, your needs, your desires, and above all, the supportive love to help you in your fight, is what you must draw towards you. Everything else is total rubbish. Your firmness in drawing in love and expelling the rest is essential to your survival. Remember you have cancer. Don't let the lesser needs of others overwhelm you as they have done in the past.

Chapter 6

AFFIRMATIONS

Positive and Negative

A smile costs nothing, but gives much. It enriches those who receive, without making poorer those who give. It takes but a moment, but the memory of it sometimes lasts forever. None is so rich or mighty that he can get along without it, and none is so poor but that he can be made rich by it. A smile creates happiness in the home, fosters goodwill in business, and is the countersign of friendship. It brings rest to the weary, cheer to the discouraged, sunshine to the sad, and it is nature's best antidote for trouble. Yet it cannot be bought, begged, borrowed or stolen, for it is something that is of no value to anyone until it is given away. Some people are too tired to give you a smile. Give them one of yours, as none needs a smile so much as he who has no more to give.
—Anon

In the last chapter we considered the love you need to identify so that you can attract it towards you, and the rest—the negativity you need to reject. As we progress through this book I am trying to encourage you to reappraise your own attitudes for your own good. Think of a tangled ball of string—just pulling at a loose end will only make the whole problem worse: the knots get tighter, the anger within you increases. You would be better to throw the string away. But that approach to the problem is negative. Consider the other way—of lovingly fingering the entire mass of string, to feel out where there is give and where there are knots. Slowly but surely (and possibly while you are getting on with something else like reading this book), you can allow your fingers to work in their own way, sorting out the string, teasing it out bit by bit like a piece of knitting in reverse. You will see this slow, sure approach is in fact a simple, caring and loving one.

You and your cancer are like that ball of string. Your fingers are the positive parts of you picking through the problem to a resolution. Think within yourself: are you like this? Are you really taking a positive and affirmative attitude to yourself, your treatment and the elimination of your cancer? Maybe you are only playing at the problem, your declaration of intent does not have that ring of assurance. In that case there is still a mass of negativity within you. Consider this carefully within yourself. I cannot place a greater importance on this aspect of your survival. There are days when I am so negative I am destroying myself and I can feel it. When the mind works on the negative levels, the body follows: my skin loses its shine, spots appear, and generally I am run down. Fears and counter-fears grow within me: "What did that mean?" I say to myself, feeling just as if a threat had been made against me or my family.

Exploring negativity

Some time ago I allowed myself to experiment to a dangerous degree with this positive versus negative attitude to my life. I wanted to prove to myself that this idea really does work. My experiment consisted of allowing a debt to arise over a period of some months. The demands for payment and settlement duly appeared followed by threats of court action and so on. On the surface I knew that I did not owe this debt. The records of the company concerned were muddled, I could see that, yet I did nothing about it. However the threats of legal action and worse troubled me, even though I knew that if the company were to spend just a few minutes with me they could see that the debt they felt I owed was in fact balanced by a credit in a similar but separate account.

Here to my mind was a good example of knowing on one level that I was without debt to the company, yet on a deeper level being upset by their threats. Dealing with a large company meant that my efforts to explain that a debt in one account was more than offset by another account in credit was frustrating and frustrated. The months passed without a solution offering itself. The threats got worse. My sleep, my whole being began to decline. I allowed this confrontation to last for 18 months until finally a debt collecting agency became involved. On sending them my file of papers they could see the problem and an apology was offered and accepted.

We are all confronted with problems of this nature, especially as society becomes less personal and more institutionalised. It is 'you' versus 'them'. This is the negative side of civilisation's progress —what is called the 'rat race'. As we are packed into tighter areas of living and working so the tensions increase. The desire for space, freedom and personal betterment occupy our minds until we reach a state of hyperactivity. Each person is unique but the stresses of modern life are a consistently negative burden on all of us. Cancer is the manifestation of an unnatural-ness or erosion of being, whatever has been the way we have sinned against our true self.

Taking the Positive Side

What we need to do is to take the positive advantages of civilisation and use them for our benefit. The problem is to know what is right for us. What is actually positive, what is actually negative? We need to try to strike a balance between these two opposing forces. If you feel that your cancer is the result of an imbalance then obviously in the short term you have to correct that. The corrections come in the ways suggested in this book: knowing your way forward in your life, being positive in your approach to treatment, diet, exercise and so on. As these factors start to have their effect on you so adjustment is needed in getting yourself in tune. For example, vitamins A and C are excellent in helping your body in its fight against cancer. If you are having chemotherapy or radiation these vitamins are par-ticularly helpful. You really can't have enough fruit and veg-etables, preferably raw. This will possibly counteract the effects of your previously less healthy diet. However, there does come a limit to just how much a body can take—even on a so-called 'healthy' diet of say carrots. Eaten in large enough quantities carrots can turn your skin carrot-coloured and your body is obviously the poorer for it. So a positive diet can, through excess, turn into a negative diet. What we are looking for is a balance of these two energies, positive and negative.

Tears and Humour

If the diet we need has to vary according to our daily requirements in a way that is neither positive nor negative but balanced, then so too do our mental needs, both emotional and intellectual. The brain is a wonder of creation. It can construct and it can destruct. My view is that it is the prime site and cause of most cancers. It is a complex structure, not unlike a computer, and quite beyond our understanding. The more we know about its workings the more we understand how little we truly know.

Right and left hemispheres

The brain is physically divided into two parts, joined in the middle by our 'decision control'. The left side of our brain is known to be our intellectual side, the right side our emotional side. In a perfectly balanced person, both sides of the brain would work equally, in perfect harmony. Possibly the central decision area would be underused in such circumstances. We are not perfect of course and our brains function according to just how much we give them to do. By nature we tend to be lazy— hence the need to go to school. School should give us the opportunity to develop both sides of our brains equally but this is rarely the case. In this society we tend to devote our energies to the intellectual or 'reasoning' side of the brain leaving the right side of the brain which involves artistic and non-logical concepts to come a poor second.

The problem we then have is that the two sides of the brain do not function at an equal level. We can and do change our minds again and again. There is therefore a fight within us between the 'trained' side of our brain and the less trained side. As relief from such problems, we have the safety valves of humour and grief, laughter and tears. Laughter is seen as a socially acceptable release of stress: grief is not. Both safety valves should in fact be used equally, as appropriate in times of need. We shouldn't laugh when others are in pain or hurt and we shouldn't grieve (another name for envy) at others' health or good luck.

Grief and loss

Bereavement is a good example of deep grieving at your own loss when you compare yourself with others who seem to be living a happy life. Having cancer is a form of bereavement. Someone considering the possibility of the removal of their breast will naturally grieve. Not only is there the operation and treatment to face, but there is the fear of disfigurement in the future. Will they lose their basic attractiveness and sexuality? How will their partners react both on the surface and inwardly towards them? Will their partner's love be strong enough to overcome this hurdle? Will in fact the love bond between them become even stronger? If that should happen then a positive good is the result.

I can say that I am glad I have had cancer. It is a unique experience. It is a battle fought within on many different levels. An excellent weapon in that fight is the ability to laugh and to cry as the need arises. As you find this out for yourself try to be aware that you will need support in these releases of stress.

Humour and laughter

See your doctor in a good humour—a joke will make him relax and open out as one human to another. Alternatively, you will be able to judge if the weight of your cancer problem is being ignored, overlooked or not dealt with as you would wish. You are frightened, depressed for yourself, your future and that of your family. At such times, tell your spouse your feelings: that you need to have a really good talk, a space to cry and to release all the fears that have accumulated within you. Find a space like a bedroom and release all that 'stuff'. The spouse should not try to get you to suppress the grief but should help the process through to a natural conclusion. Raging and beating out this inner anger is good and healthy.

Such a period of grief should last no more than half an hour. Once you have got the rubbish out of your system you feel better. You should not be in any way embarrassed by the strength of your emotional outburst. Once you are free of these negative emotions you will recognise an overall improvement in your being. If you leave the anger and grief to ferment within you, then you will release small outbursts at your friends, snap at your family, constantly driving them away from you by your negative attitudes. This leads to inner and real loneliness, something which many cancer patients discover, causing further unhappiness and depression. There is no future along that way and your back must be firmly turned against such attitudes.

Toxins

When I was a small boy, like all small boys, I naturally had sulks —and oh were they powerful! At such times of moody feelings my mother would tell me to walk round the block of houses in London where we lived. I suppose the walk was no more than a third of a mile, perhaps less. I dared not disobey my parents so I would set off, still in a thoroughly resentful mood which I gamely tried to maintain. I succeeded until about 100 steps from home. At that moment the mood would evaporate. Hard as I tried, I could no longer hold it. As a result of the combination of exercise, self contemplation and the chance to see what a little wretch I was, I was able to say "I am sorry", and I would be embraced in forgiveness. What a magic moment that was—all the past bad mood was forgotten.

During such moments of depression our body is full of toxins, poisons that need to be eliminated. On a physical level, you can get rid of these toxins through exercise and working up a good healthy sweat. Think of the times you go swimming—your mind is perhaps full of things you must do. Think of the times you leave swimming—your mind has forgotten these things you must do. Toxins are constantly within your body, and if harboured in areas of inactivity they tend to create problems. Toxins in the cancer medicine you may be having will also cause problems if they are not eliminated from your system as quickly as possible. The medicine has to do its duty but then it must be got rid of promptly. See that you do this effectively.

If you are in bed, consider the importance of moving all the toxic wastes within you. Take suitable action in going to the toilet many times. If you can get out of bed, so much the better. Walk up and down as often as you can—all exercise at times of illness is important if you truly want to get well. Allowing your bowels to be constipated will prevent fresh food from being assimilated and will allow the toxins to accumulate. This means a double negative on a physical level and you certainly won't be happy within your mind either.

So the cancer battle is fought around the lavatory. The purity of your food and drink and good exercise will eliminate the toxins on a daily basis. Some treatments for cancer of the bowel involve the use of coffee enemas. The coffee is seen as an effective purge and much useful help is given in what is called the Gerson Therapy.

A reminder

I trust that you are still marking the margin of this book with a pencil, underlining key passages and recording suitable passages in your diary. Am I nagging you as a parent might? Yes? Good, that is the intention! Like my mother who told me to walk round the block, so I am at times telling you to do something similar, to give you the space to clear yourself. Go on, you can do it. At other times I will draw you close to my heart. You are truly sorry? Then you are truly forgiven. Your faith will make you whole.

Yoga

"Cancer" is a spine-chilling word and I came face to face with it at a recent yoga seminar I attended. I laid down my mat and sat there waiting for the session to start. To my left was the pale figure of a man deep in meditation; his "spirit-like" being intrigued my mind. He was later introduced as Colin Ryder Richardson who was to give a lecture during the afternoon on the holistic approach to cancer.

I spoke to him a little during lunch about his diet. I perhaps expected it to be a very strict regime but it consisted of fresh, natural foods with very little meat. He could "feel" which foods were his.

Colin played soft music all the while he was talking. He had found harmony of mind, body and spirit through yoga. He knew only too well that the power to overcome this "disease of disharmony" was within himself. Cancer was a gift—the sufferer begins to re-assess himself and revalue his life. Colin believes that cancer is a build up of stress, fear and tension that cannot naturally be got rid of. The "cancer person" was an uncomplaining, accepting type. I translated this to mean a repressive, negative type, sometimes the type of person we would think of as kind. It seems that we all have the ability to destroy ourselves. When Colin discovered he had cancer it was a major step in his evolution; he now rejoices. It took a crisis for him to look inside himself to discover his own needs and understand his emotions.

Colin did in fact have surgery to remove his stomach, took the prescribed drugs and had chemotherapy. Through meditation he encouraged these drugs to heal his body. Through yoga he had learned that positive belief in what he was doing was powerful enough to help him—mind over matter. When we accept life we accept that death is a part of it—disease is capable of ending our life span in a too abrupt manner. We are not prepared. Cancer is a way of telling us that we are on the wrong path.

Through yoga Colin has become aware of his higher spiritual existence—love emanates from every pore in his body. He no longer passes on the responsibility for his well being to others, he has taken over sole responsibility for his own peace.

There must be many paths to self realisation and the cancer sufferer must find whichever is right for him. Our society, packed with wars, riots and crime, is suffering from cancer in desperate need of union, love and peace.

As I walked out into the day I was very aware of the disharmony in my own life and of the conscious effort needed to create the necessary balance.

Sylvia Jean Sheppard, *a yoga student*

It is said that when someone is ready for yoga, the teacher will appear. Also that when someone is ready to teach yoga, the students will appear. You may ask why the subject of yoga comes up in such a book as this. My view is that a person who correctly practises yoga will find that its disciplines help him or her to fight cancer on all levels. One (cancer, which equals imbalance) is the the precise opposite of the other (yoga, which equals balance).

This view is not just my own, but one shared by a large number of people. The latest medical books devote whole sections to yoga for the benefits it brings. Medical organisations recommend that in combating stress and other self-induced degenerative diseases, certain yogic practises are followed regularly. Evidence is growing that people who regularly practise yoga live longer, are healthier, happier, and become more excellent in their way of life. Those who wish to rise above average find that yoga helps them do this. Those who are less well or who are handicapped find similar benefit.

So what is this yoga? It is a life discipline involving body, mind and spirit. It is not a religion. It works on the improvement of the body in slow physical movements and this in turn extends to the opening of the mind in awareness. The combination of the two enhances the spirit. Yoga is practised all over the country.

Small groups meet regularly on a weekly basis and a village hall is a typical location. All you need is loose clothing and a mat for floor work. Before doing the exercises you should not have eaten for at least two hours.

If you can truly say that your cancer is the result of a build-up of stress, that the knowledge of your disease has caused further stress, that you can't sleep and are worried sick by all the problems that suddenly seem to have landed on your shoulders, then yoga is your answer. By now you may have realised that my advice to help yourself is not going to be easy to follow. On the contrary, it will be hard, very hard. It will be like running a long distance. There will be barriers and hurdles which you think you cannot surmount. However, you can. You can do anything if you really set your mind to do it.

Turning around that negative energy of 'can't' to 'can' is all a matter of mental attitude. OK, so no excuses. There are many yoga classes near you and the cost is minimal. Anyway, who is counting cost if you are going to get better as I did? "Colin, how do I get to know a good teacher?" That is easy. A good teacher is one to whom you will wish to return time and time again to learn more. Such a teacher will have a fair number of other students and it might be difficult to get in. You should arrive early and explain your medical problems and if necessary tell your doctor what you intend to do so that you can obtain his clearance and approval. He will undoubtedly confirm that going to a yoga class is perfectly OK unless there is some temporary problem such as a recent operation.

The yoga class

A yoga class generates a magic quality of love. Students arrive in an animated state of mind, cross the threshold and find that calmness and tranquility begin to manifest themselves into a peace without boundaries. The whole becomes greater than the sum of its parts. Trying to describe the quality of a yoga class is impossible. You have to go and do and experience. At the end of the class, students seem to 'float' out in an inner serenity that is vital to them. A teacher will encourage the students to retain this inspirational quality within them until at least the next time.

Every teacher is unique in the way he or she teaches so is every student in learning. When I attended my first class as a middle-aged, highly tense, overweight individual I saw immediately that yoga was beautiful, graceful and not just for women but for everybody. For years I had longed to take part in sports but my physical problems with my veins prevented this. Here at last was an activity that was non-competitive, could be practised in the simplest way possible and was highly beneficial in restoring one's balance in all things.

The physical class is the first step. Almost as soon as you learn about moving your body slowly and surely in the stretches, twists and balances, you also learn of the effects it has on calming the mind. As your practise expands so does your awareness of how little you know, and how much you want to know. It is like living in one room in a palace. Suddenly you have the keys to so many doors. The doors lead to rooms of splendour, to gardens of intense beauty. Your life suddenly expands in the freedom of love. No longer are you a prisoner of your self, your physical and mental abilities reach out like a kite soaring in the sky. Yoga is beautiful and breath-taking.

Do not expect immediate benefits. Your cancer, your stress, has taken time to manifest itself, so you must allow the reversal of your former self to take time to obtain benefits. You may be in bed thinking how can yoga help me—but it can. I have given a class where technically it was possible to do all the work within such a limited area. Imagine you have a rusty bicycle in a garden shed. It was yours many years ago but it has been neglected. You wheel it out, clean it, oil it, repair what is necessary and pump up the tyres. Suddenly you are rather proud of the time and effort you have spent and the reward is that your familiar old bicycle is renewed. You ride off in victory and relearn your old skills of riding and stopping. Now you can turn that useless junk into an object of use. It can take you to far away places for pleasure, for work, to make new friends, or just to expand your awareness of the world that all the time has existed around you.

You, yes you—*your* body is that bicycle. Yoga is the energy that can turn 'junk' into something of value. The body improves, old skills are re-awakened and new frontiers are crossed. Others can help but only you can ride and achieve. So go ride your bike.

Prayer

Prayer is the mental desire for assistance from within. Through prayer we seek spiritual guidance for our past misdeeds, our present needs, and guidance for the future. We can direct our prayer to help others as well as ourselves. To pray is to ask for a way forward. Yogis believe that if you honestly ask for something then it will come about. Not perhaps quite in the way you had expected but nevertheless requests truly made will be answered. But prayer can be the directing of energies towards death. Many feel that cancer is just such a manifestation—"I wish I were dead"; "I wish so and so was dead". Such words horrify others who respond that such thoughts should be denied. All that is necessary is to redirect this negative energy into a positive affirmation.

At every level I find that those with cancer have expressed these intensely negative prayers. These negative prayers are undoubtedly being answered like a form of suicide. Ask and it shall be given. Unfortunately, when the prayer wish is actually being fulfilled there is a cry for help. In many cases, it is too late. Already the last process is in action like a supertanker whose forward movement onto the rocks cannot be reversed.

If it all seems inevitable then surely prayer or any action is useless? That is the heart of the cancer problem. Just how committed are you to reversing the process? How inevitable is your case? Prayer can be directed towards a new you with a new committed attitude to cast off the old ways. Just how strongly and honestly your prayers come from the inner being will be how seriously you take advice for your health. Take treatment—people say to me that such and such a treatment will cost too much—is there anything cheaper, easier, even free! Frankly they put a price on their own future. It is for them to decide what they truly can afford in terms of time, money and effort. Starting to pray can clear one's mind so that what is important to you comes to the surface.

Love

Thou art the sun and the moon
Thou art the stars that twinkle in the dark'ning sky
Thou art the seed that waits within a mother's womb
The dew that rests upon the thirsty ground
Thou art my heart's blood and my every thought—
the way my feet would tread—given the strength
Thou art my strength
The stillness of my heart . . .
The tender blossom in a baby's hand
Thou art the nectar for my thirsting soul
The hand that leads me thro' life's tortuous ways
Thou art my treasure and my heart's delight
Thou art my all,
Thou art,
Thou
Art . . .

— Patti

Love is the coming together of two mutual energies. This book is directed and dedicated in love from one with cancer to another. I hope that in return your feelings are beginning to respond towards me in equal warmth. Love is an essential ingredient in a book of this nature. Our holding hands on our journey turns into hugs of love. Why should this be so? Because cancer is everything that love is not. Cancer is chaos, like an inner explosion of the body intent on changing and destroying. The inner panics and fears release the adrenalin over and over again until our immune system collapses and allows the cancer to grow in our weakest part. It starts in a primary site and may well move on to a secondary area. Cancer is wholly unpredictable and must be fought on every level. Love is the greatest help because it abounds within everything around. All we need to do is to tap into it. I love my wife Rosemary, my family, my friends, my pets, but do I love myself—the most important person in my life? This question you must ask yourself. We all need to confront it and to be honest in our responses. Then write your answer large in your diary on a daily basis.

Love of the self

If you love yourself, will you feed the foods that you know are good for you? Or will you go on eating any old rubbish? Will you seek out those things that can help you and reject those that can't? Will you take the treatment because you know that it is the right course although you may not wish to? Do you not realise that love is manifold; to deny yourself something that you should accept will not only affect you but all those who love you. Can you receive love unconditionally as I offer it?

Time and time again I learn of how love has brought a better understanding through the fire of cancer, that the quality of life has improved because the shock of cancer has made someone realise how lucky they have been. Rosemary my wife has fought the fight with me—shoulder to shoulder. As lovers, like soldiers, finding the way forward hand in hand so that our love has been tested in and out of hospital. This has meant that we have really both had cancer because we shared all pain and problems together in an inspirational way. We are not alone, many others have found this way forward, and have found that love conquers all. It fights the barriers put up by the institutions and their servants. It fights the "sorry, we can't help" brigade, and it fights the desperation deep within our selves.

Chapter 7

VISUALISATIONS

The Workings of the Mind

Shyam Meditation Hermitage
Valley of Gods
Himalayas
Kulu HP
India

Dearest Colin,

I received your letter and it delighted me. I came to know the facts about your work and what you are doing. God works in mysterious ways: He cured your cancer so that you may be interested in curing further cancers and that's fine work. If you want that deaths may not increase due to cancer, then introduce meditation in the life of the patient and the lives of those not yet the patients of cancer. It is difficult work but the cure is sure. So add meditation in your program. Read the book "Why Meditation" thoroughly, study it, and be a great liberator of the man from death's destruction.

I enjoyed Rosemary's letter very much, she's doing well. Tell her whenever she finds time and it is in time with God's will, we will meet. Till then we remember each other in the space through letters. I thank the blessed moment when we met.

With love,
Your own self,

Shyam

We have touched briefly on yoga and love and these two energies find their source in the mind. You may have seen yogis who through mind control can walk without harm on hot beds of coals. I do not approve of such practises and don't suggest you try them but they do show the strength that can be generated by putting mind above matter. You may know people who so love another that when they lose that partner, in their loss, they find love has disappeared out of their lives. Maybe you are such a person?

Both these aspects of our mind show just how strong it is when properly put to work. One method of mind control is visualisation. Visualisation is in fact an active form of meditation or prayer. You should select a quiet place—say your bedroom—and ensure that you are not disturbed. Your yoga teacher may instruct you on how to meditate. It is simple, relaxing and should be done twice a day. In essence you sit quietly in your chosen place and allow yourself to come into touch with your inner self. You try to envisage your cancer, where it is in your body, what damage has been done, whether it is getting smaller or bigger, what has caused it in the first place and what you are going to do to get rid of it.

Place your hands over the affected area and mentally try to picture what is going on within. At the same time take in the thought that your treatment is having an effect in its battle with the cancer cells. Your treatment is also having a positive effect on your body's immune system. These if you like are the good forces within you, repelling the negative invaders. It is a battle of survival so try to be aware that through the energy in your hands and fingers you are directing extra energy to fight that battle in your favour.

Some people imagine their cancer as a nest of snakes and the forces directed to get rid of them as the keepers in a zoo. One by one the keepers return those snakes to their proper place back in the jungle. It does not matter what imagery you use provided you can identify the two forces of evil and good in the battle within you. It is also useful to superimpose an outline of your 'cancer' on a diagram of your body. Keep this in your diary; it will help you concentrate during the exercise above. The more often you do these visualisation exercises the better—in this way you can begin to get in closer touch with your problem.

Meditation should take place as part of your daily yoga practise. Try to meditate twice a day, first thing in the morning and during the evening. The use of the active visualisation technique needs practise and personal advice. At first you may feel foolish but soon you will learn how such work can have an effect. So don't doubt, just get to work and channel the energy of good to the places most needed within you. Although visualisation is a more active form of meditation less active methods are equally valuable.

Meditation is always carried out in a quiet place, somewhere that is comfortable and warm. It is something which should be enjoyed by your innermost being. Practising some yoga movements before you meditate can help when you are a beginner. However ill you are you can always breathe. Learning how to breathe in a yogic way is important because you find out just how slight and shallow are the breaths you take in everyday life.

The value of breath

Yogis believe that in breathing you inhale an energy which is called *prana*, or the life force. It is the essential form of life energy and it is found in air, water, sun, food, drink—and love. Taking these within you in their purest form and converting them into life energy is part of yogic practice. Learning to breathe more deeply of the purest air available helps your body enormously. This is why smoking is so bad for us because you are denying your body an essential fuel and filling your body with toxins.

In order to meditate properly you need to bring yourself into a harmonious balance through some simple yogic movements and yoga breathing exercises. Even if you are confined to your bed you can always find someone who will teach you to breathe correctly. The basis is this: as you sit quietly breathing in and out, mentally repeat a sequence of words or a phrase to calm down your mind. Some useful phrases are 'I breathe in, I breathe out', 'I take in the good, I expel the waste'. Whatever words you find right for you are the words you should use.

How to meditate

Each meditation session (normally carried out in a quiet place), should last 20 minutes. At first it is difficult, your mind constantly pops from subject to subject. If this worries you during meditation then use your diary to write down all the vexing matters that are interrupting you; list the lot. Now try again. No noise should disturb you—as you meditate a serenity should start to pervade your innermost self.

Sit comfortably, eyes shut, hands relaxed, body relaxed and warm. Just sit quietly. Now listen to your breath—concentrate only on your breath. Just allow your mind to select the form of meditation you wish to enjoy. The only thing to keep in mind is that the meditation, whatever form it takes, will be for your good. Perhaps the meditation will be on visualising or perhaps it will be simply concentrating on a beautiful garden or some other beautiful image that you bring to mind. Thinking yourself positively into a place of beauty can be difficult to start with. You may be restless, may feel you are wasting time. You hear a telephone and your mind wanders. Gently bring your mind back to the chosen form of your meditation. Remember that the meditation that is good for me is not necessarily the one that is good for you. You are unique. Your mind is unique. You are asking your mind to slow down (not to stop) but to devote all energy to a subject of natural beauty. Suddenly you will find doors in your mind open, matters long forgotten will come to the surface, bringing perhaps tears, perhaps happiness. Allow this to happen as this is a stress being released—perhaps a matter you had totally forgotten about in your 'everyday' mind. However, deep down, there it was, waiting for permission to surface. Meditation gives that permission through release.

Just imagine a pond. You are that pond. The ripples of the wind stir that pond. Pebbles cast into that pond cause other ripples, crossing and re-crossing each other. Follow down the pebbles as they sink to the bottom—into the thick mud that has accumulated over time. An energy within the mud begins to stir, just like bubbles of gas forming. More and more bubbles form and come together until there is enough strength for the bubbles to rise towards the pond's surface. If these thought bubbles find a calm surface you will find you can identify and deal with them. But if the pond is stirred by waves of emotion, the bubbles create an even greater upset until there is a seething ferment from above and below. This is the cancerous state which we are trying to avoid. We are seeking a calmness both on the surface and within our selves.

Meditating with others is helpful, and if you can share your experiences and lead one another into ways of improving your meditation then this is better still. The best arrangement is to find a skilled teacher and discover if the methods taught are good for you. It is all part of your self discovery. No one way is better than another. We all seek the best, but the benefits are only found along the path of self discovery.

Stillness

Be still
Be aware of the Spirit of you
Hear the sounds of nature around
Understand compassion
Love one another
Find the essence within everything
Forgive yourself
Everything passes
See the oneness within everything
Understand the harmony
Be aware of the balance
Feel the spine growing
Now
See the spirit of you within
Know your gifts
Find your own message
Radiate your being
Radiate everything
Accept it all
Be still
Everything passes
Be aware of the Spirit of you
Loving opens everything
— Peace (Frances, 'Quiet Waters', Scotland)

Drawing Upon the Inner Energy

The greatest common factor of cancer patients is a feeling of being alone, insecure, frightened, panicked and lacking the will to go on. It is as if the plug has been pulled out of the bath water of life and all the energy is draining away so fast. Almost with morbid fascination the cancer patient can tell when it is that the water of life will drain out and there is nothing they can do or even want to do. To them it is inevitable and they even seem to try to hasten this negative withdrawal of life's inner energy. Even the most loving of family support cannot do anything. If anything it seems to make matters worse. Self pity, a feeling of 'leave me alone', a lack of any will to do anything are common cancer attitudes.

It is important to know that these panics are common—as common as spots with measles. It is part of the disease of the mind. The 'I don't want to live', the 'Why should it happen to me?' and all the other thousand and one negative excuses. Record all your negative reasons and then laugh at them for they are absurd. Mock them and cast them behind you. Even if you do not truly believe in this mental exercise do it for the sake of those you love. Just mock these villains in your mind to scorn. Listen instead to the wisdom of the child and learn to be reborn.

You must know that in coming to terms with cancer we have to realise that we have mentally dropped a long way down a well of despair. No longer are you at the top—you are down at the bottom of a hole. Very well, you must say, this is a reverse which will need a fresh cunning to overcome and you will need to draw on your inner energy to climb back out of the well. The inner energy is located in the centre of yourself. You may feel totally hollow. Meditation and other yogic techniques will open up your centre to an energy which we have already discussed: *prana*. When you still the overactive mind and feed on the pranic energy of breath, food, water, sun and love, you will replete your centre.

Finding new energy

As you begin to enjoy pure energy flowing into your centre so you can draw on that energy to smile and open out in all ways. This is difficult to describe because the energy appears in different ways to different people. You might for instance decide to write to a long lost friend and find this act to be a very simple but basic step in the right direction. Suddenly you have time to do this. Whatever the action or thought is, just recognise it as a positive act. That positive act, however slight, is good. It means a drawing out of your innermost reserves, it is a positive affirmation on which can be built more and more such acts until your life is totally, totally changed. This is your inner crucifixion. The change from the negative way to the positive way. Know now that at that point in your life things will improve.

Naturally there will be downs again, but finding the way up becomes simpler because you have done it before and you can do it again if your will is there to do it. This is if you like the centre of this book. Up till now we have collected ourselves together, identified the problems, decided on courses of action, directed our energies and become aware of new possibilities in our return to health so as to assist our doctors in their task. At this juncture we start to climb out of the well of despair, to expand, to walk along our path with an air of confidence in our health, our future and happiness. Our energy is lubricated in love and we are at one with ourselves. Mind you, we still have a long way to go and we are still weak, so our first positive steps need plenty of reinforcement.

For Colin

Unshutter all the pain
Release the tension and the strife
Keep ever in your consciousness
The sacredness of life
Hold ever in your mind
The power of love you have to give
And in your giving find
The overwhelming need to live

Be therefore of more tranquil mind
Seek out the peaceful state
Within yourself, and thus in love
A greater love create

87

To shine forth like the lotus pattern's
Love and thus forgive
And in forgiving find
The overwhelming need to live

Be thus at peace within yourself
And with the world outwith
Reach out to love your fellow man
In oneness, kin and kith
And 'heal thyself' will thus become
The healing love you give
To all mankind in peace
The overwhelming will to live

— John McLeod, 1.15pm, 28 May 1982, Stansted.

Healing

When I was very, very ill with cancer and still suffering from the aftermath of my operation and chemotherapy I felt extremely sorry for myself. I seemed to be a frightened prisoner in my body awaiting the release of death. How often have I seen that. Not only in people but in baby rabbits caught by a cat. The rabbit appears to be unharmed but if one picks it up it lies terrifies in one's hand, its eyes distant, its body silent except for maintenance breathing. Such a small creature is only a blink away from death. Yet it still lives and like the rabbit, the cure can lie in our very own hands, depending on our own abilities and also on the strength of will of the rabbit. These two energies must come together to give the best chance of life.

Dottie Hook is a healer and along with Greta Gill and many, many friends—too many to name—gave me regular healing. To them I owe my life and I thank them for their love. When I was ill, at first I was too weak to protest at this army of people who came to the house, not to sympathise at my illness, but to offer healing. It seemed to me at that time to be a form of black magic but I could not protest, only watch from my inner prison. It was as if in a dream that hands touched me and love surrounded me.

At first I was angry—where had they got my permission to do this. Rosemary did not stand any of this negativity so I resigned myself to accepting the inevitable. 'It can't do any good but it can't do any harm either and anyway after a few weeks they will lose interest in me' was what I thought—a stupid assessment.

Still the healers came, and still come, years later, to offer a form of love which is so wholesome and good that I wonder now how I could have thought of rejecting such healing. This just shows how negative a person can be. Are you like this? Be honest. As week followed week the healing continued, under the active encouragement of Rosemary. Frankly I felt I was getting better or worse depending on where I was with my chemotherapy treatment. What I did not notice was that while I did slide back to the bottom, the inner energy discussed earlier allowed me to climb back up again, perhaps a little higher than before. I only seemed to notice how ill I was—the negative parts. Dottie would continue to appear, especially if I was very low. Her regular visits were encouraging to me but I did not feel she and her healing were actually actively helping me. I was still not converted, not convinced, little realising that I was beginning to be more of a normal person and less of a living corpse.

Once I began to look back over my diary for this period, I began to see my progress and my *conversion* to the benefits of healing was total. Soon I was meeting other healers who also had this quality of giving and sharing, of being concerned and loving towards the sick. Healing is a natural energy that we all need. When you hurt your body, you cover the hurt with a hand. A child falls and is engulfed in the healing of the mother's embrace. A cancer patient is looking for such love, the warm genuine embrace of a good friend to another. Sometimes a family cannot provide this very basic form of help and so healers are essential to comfort and console and to direct healing energy or prana to the inner self.

I feel good after a session of healing. That is as it should be, nothing more, nothing less. Just love from someone who cares to someone who needs love. It is like coming home to rest. Some healers can direct their love over distances in what is called absent healing. A group can form to channel their energy in thoughts towards a patient who is absent. In a way this is a form of prayer. If the patient is open to receive such prayer, then much good will follow. From this one can see that prayer through religious practise, and healing, form part of a natural chain of activity. My great regret is that religions seem in general to have overlooked this. Religion has gone one way, medical practise another and the gap in the middle is where we find ourselves.

Looking Into Nature

Each step of civilisation takes us further from natural life. I love the benefits of modern life and I can't wait for what the future will bring. However, we forget our natural past and this brings problems. Men and women lead artificial lives which they may enjoy for many years, little seeing that they can build up big problems within themselves. We are not meant to live a life of stress, of rushing on regardless of our own basic needs and those of others. We are meant to use our bodies and not let machines do all the lifting, carrying, washing, even entertaining (look at the role of television and radio).

We are meant to be doers and not watchers like the many thousands of watchers at a football match. We should not be burned out by stressful work by the age of 30, or even 40 or later. We should know that certain pains are warnings and should not suppress them with drugs. We should enjoy life in a balanced and natural way and those of us who are prepared to listen, learn, and do, will find the discipline they need through yoga.

So here I am saying that I look forward to the future benefits of civilisation but at the same time I am rubbishing the benefits that are available. Yoga teaches us to use all energy in a balanced way. I use my car to take me to a park where I can walk for my benefit. I would not like to use a car in place of this walking. I enjoy television to entertain and instruct but not when it stays switched on all hours of the day and night. I call this kind of television moving wallpaper.

In a similar way I have allowed modern medicine and surgery to assist in my cancer treatment but once the crisis is over I improve my own wellbeing by natural forms of healing. So civilisation and nature can go hand in hand as long as we keep that control of knowing that a bit of each will keep us in balance. We do not want to be a rubbish tip of stresses as a result of too much civilisation, nor do we want to be a hermit who dies of cold as a result of too much nature.

The natural way

Nature has many effective cures for our body. The greatest are our own built-in systems such as the immune system. Yogic practices help to strengthen such systems in ways well beyond our present understanding. Modern civilised man without nature can look old at twenty. A yogi can look youthful at eighty. Why? A foolish modern youth has the benefit of a beautiful body which can resist certain abuses. So the foolish youth goes further and the course of nature is diverted by these excessive acts. A yogi does the opposite and is aware of the strength of nature and uses that strength for his or her benefit.

Natural benefits extend into natural medicines and these can prove effective provided they are expertly prescribed and correctly taken. Notes on such medicines are given on page 46. A placebo is a preparation that has no known medical powers. But if a placebo is effective does it not follow that we do not yet fully understand the whole workings of our body? Perhaps a placebo works because no drug effect is induced and the normal bodily healing powers are allowed to come into play. Healing could be considered to be a placebo—if so I would prescribe it for you. It gives you time to relax, to sort out your inner self. Allow your body to take charge rather than you.

The Daily Routine

Your normal daily routine probably involves serving others in some way and excluding yourself. That has to change. You are now the most important person in your life—you have cancer, so you have a priority and no stresses should come between you and getting better. When I was very ill I made sure I had deep sleep several times every 24 hours, deep meditation, short periods of activity, constant pure natural food and drink and a burning desire to get out and about. I used my wife and friends to give me help in any way they offered it and I am so very thankful they were able to assist me.

Now that I am so much better my life is very full from 6am to 11pm daily. I rise at six, do some simple yogic stretches, wash, dress and prepare my breakfast. I eat several rounds of brown bread and honey (no butter) and drink a weak tea, sometimes herbal depending on my mood. I meditate and having taken tea to Rosemary, leave on my motorcycle for work at a few minutes after seven. The journey to the city is 30 miles and during that time I come to terms with myself, preparing for work at about eight.

Normally I have nuts and dried fruit by me at work so that I can maintain a constant flow of good food. During the day I am aware of the tensions that build up within me—when schedules are not met, targets not reached. Each time I note my anxiety rise and take such steps as I can to counteract these stresses. Usually I succeed but sometimes I don't. What I do know is that I do not want to repeat my compoundingly terrible pre-cancer stresses. To come home tired out, irritable with myself and family, wondering where all my efforts were getting me—it seemed they were getting me further in the mud, into total confusion, tiredness and despair. A family with hungry mouths to feed can rob you of all energy. We can be our own worst enemy and this was me. All my energy was misdirected.

I then took up yoga and found a total change and a new energy as I have already described. Now when I leave work at about four to five-thirty I am not exhausted. On the contrary I am filled with the pleasure in store of riding home and taking part in Rosemary's yoga and aerobics classes. So I get home, have a real change, bath, relaxation, meditation, then off to two evening classes on three nights of the week. On other evenings I may be seeing friends, counselling or writing (this book, for example). My life is full and enjoyable. Each step I take, even each thought, is carefully handled. I weigh my actions to ensure that I get the greatest personal benefit in the most economical means and with the least stress.

My friends are most important. They must also be Rosemary's friends so that they are truly *our* friends and in whose company I can be totally relaxed. My friends understand my eating needs, my aversion to smoking and so on. I see no need to tolerate other people's social ill manners in matters such as smoking in no smoking areas. Now I will speak my mind and ask people to stop because I have cancer. It usually works.

My days end with a quiet period, perhaps with the lights out in bed to quieten down the turmoil in my mind from the day's events. In this way dreams are few and pleasant because my 'computer' brain has dumped its load of stuff. You will note that my daily routine puts my self first. If I forget myself, how can I be prepared to help others? This book for example and writing it does not become the ogre in my life but the servant of my thoughts for our betterment. I hope you are becoming in tune with these thoughts for your own good.

Music

> In the beginning was the word (the sound, the light?)
> — *John 1.1*

Music can uplift and inspire or it can irritate and depress. We do not appreciate just how easily we can be influenced by music. It seems natural to me now that a person whose mind is stressed and in a turmoil can be quietly calmed if the right music is played. Knowing the right piece is part of the problem but once you find music that provides a satisfactory quietening of your hyperactivities then that should be your theme. Our evening classes are filled with music, the aerobics classes with a beat that is in time to the physical movements. It is infectious and fun and that is as it should be. The yoga classes have music that lulls and which provides tranquility of mind. In all classes the students come into harmonic tune and oneness with each other. When we are born music is the sound of the beat of your mother's heart. This satisfactory rhythm of life is the focal point of a baby's existence. What we should be looking for is a continuous harmonic flow in our life that we find acceptable. This should flood our being to suit our needs. Our liberty should not be invaded by noises that are discordant and gross. Stillness in meditation is one of the more subtle melodies and should ensure that your space is properly filled with the sounds you love.

You should try to become a more private and selective person in the matter of the sounds that surround you. If this is difficult then move to where you know that you will enjoy what you hear. The same applies to all aspects of your life. Look for absence of discord. Ask yourself these questions:

Are your friends upsetting you?
Are your past experiences upsetting you?
Are you happy with your life?
Are you feeling a loss?
Are you eating and drinking only what is good for you?
Do you love your spouse or close companion and the way they love you?
Do you love your family?
Do you now know what has been a discord in your life?
Have you failed?
Are you expected to do more than you can?
Would you relive your life the way it was?
Do you know the cause or causes of your cancer?
Are you guilty?
What are your guilts?

In other words has your life been in harmony with you. Just meditate on these questions and see how truthfully you can answer. Notice where you lie even to yourself. Be true to thine own self and learn to sing your song of life.

Chapter 8

DEDICATIONS

The Will

We have already passed the centre of this book but we are not yet half-way. We are really at the beginning and always shall be. Life stretches out ahead of us as a path. The longer the life, the longer the path. This thought might depress you but you should convert that negativity into a positive flow of energy.

How? By finding the will, the determination that the path ahead will be better in quality than that which has already passed. A cancer crisis brings one into a jumble of fears and panics. When you see your doctor his or her words are lost; life seems to have dealt you a rotten blow; you are filled with regrets, fears, angers, lies. Even reading this book is a gross imposition. "He doesn't know how I feel", you say. But I do.

You are not unique in your negative feelings. You will not get better if you maintain those feelings. In fact I can assure you you will get worse. Your mind is very powerful and if you feel you are going to die, you will. It is as simple as that. If you feel that inner anger is eating you up then the cancer you have is doing exactly that. Yes the doctors can possibly cut out the cancer or kill it with medicine but what is to stop the cancer reappearing some time later? So we are always at the beginning, in the now. Don't let that thought depress you. Just know that you cannot allow the ghosts of the past to haunt you now and for the future. Cancer is the time of change for the better for you. It is a time for the unlocking of the shackles of the past and the stepping gently but firmly onto a new path forward. All is change and now you should be beginning to feel it.

The will to learn from past mistakes, to preserve your present being and to look eagerly into the future lies within you. Sit and meditate on this. Quietly, the correct solution to the way you move forward will emerge. The method of your recovery will start with allowing the will to generate. It does not have to be in gross physical activity—that might lead to despair. It might be in learning to say 'yes' instead of 'no' or 'no' instead of 'yes'. There is no room for 'maybe' or any of those similar 'mights' or 'think about it' thoughts.

The will means actual determination of what will be done by *you* regardless of other people's suggestions—even mine. All I can do is point the way. You have to generate the will within you and it is there I assure you.

Listening to Your Body and Mind

We discussed music which is the art of listening only to what you wish to hear or not hear. Now we consider the aspects of your body and mind. Just look at your body in a mirror. Forget those silly opinions you have formed about it. Consider instead its sheer beauty of form. Know that it is composed of thousands of millions of cells that are normally actively being born, living and dying. It is governed, policed, fed, nurtured and disposed in much the same way as a nation or a people. We can therefore consider your body as a nation of individuals going about their everyday activities.

To a greater or lesser extent the individual cell, the person, is just one of many millions without importance. Provided the cell/person abides by the natural laws then harmony prevails. Sometimes problems occur and the police immune system steps in, takes suitable action and life returns to normal. However, if the nation/body is going through a period of difficulties a change begins to evolve. This may mean unemployment, strikes, riots, depression, and similar developments. Perhaps the problems are caused by malnutrition, or a monotonous diet of the same over-rich foods lacking in vital energy, or perhaps doses of acrid tobacco smoke which pervade every pore of the whole nation/body. At times like this the cell/individual that creates the problem finds others who feel the same. They band together in a determination of chaotic destruction. The growth of this chaos spreads and the police are unable to contain the problem. The location of the outbreak becomes a 'no go' area. Suddenly the host body is confronted by an internal revolution that has no fixed ideas or aims except the total destruction of established order. So shops, homes, factories are burnt, looted and destroyed and chaos expands.

Bad news travels fast and almost as soon as the government/ brain begins to realise the size of the disaster, the other areas of body/nation begin to react in sympathy to the primary area. These are the secondary growth areas and it is amazing to note the similarity of the way cancer can react and spread to the way an internal riot can affect first one city then others and finally the government. History books are full of such examples.

Our mind/government has now had the shock news that cancer has broken out in an area. Existing immune police systems have been unable to contain the problem and reports of growing areas of chaos are gradually filtering through. Like all governments the mind is slow to react, perhaps the reports are *exaggerated*. Even if they are true perhaps after the weekend the situation will be under control. Unfortunately the reports are only about mild problems and finally when the mind/government determines upon outside help, matters may already be very serious.

Outside help to contain the outbreak now consists of a task force of surgeons and chemists who will cut out, poison, irradiate and if possible totally destroy the known affected areas. So peace is restored. How long do we have that peace? Has the government/brain determined itself on a set of reforms? Has it got the will of the people again? Are they being loved, properly fed and employed and motivated towards a better future? Look at your body and self and allow this lesson to be constantly with you.

Counselling

It takes courage to call for outside help. There are plenty of books such as this one but personal counselling is essential. We are all unique. Some of us truly want to live, others don't. Which are you? Well, you have got this far in the book. But the journey for your future is still on the starting line. You need the help of an outsider or outsiders who have no axe to grind, no special therapies up their sleeves, who are open to hear your problems and to advise you from the heart of their experience. Always the decision is yours but you need to know what is available for you.

I get many calls and letters asking for help and this I gladly give. It helps me as much as it helps the cancer sufferer. I recognise that each call for help is an act of courage often from a spouse who is sometimes more distraught than the patient. I always ask if the cancer sufferer really wants to see me and I satisfy myself on this point. It is important to know this because this represents the person's will to get better, to fight the battle and win through at all costs.

Incidentally, I make no charge for counselling as I feel this gets in the way of the truth. Like you I never meant to get cancer. That happens to others doesn't it? However, once you appear to have overcome your cancer problem then the news will spread and you will be drawn as I have been into offering help to others. This is how the cancer self help groups network spreads across the world. I would strongly recommend that you join your local group and details can easily be obtained from hospitals or local authorities or perhaps your local paper. All these cancer self help groups provide a holistic back-up service to complement your medical treatment. You are therefore getting help in two ways: the holistic way of gentle love, care, advice and direction, and the medical way. The choice is yours to opt for either or both.

What happens in counselling

When I get a call it goes something like this: "I wonder if you can help—my husband (wife) has been told he (she) has cancer. We are at our wits end and we are very frightened." Naturally I ask if the husband (wife) really wants to see me. Usually I ask to speak to him (her) if he (she) is well enough and possibly I drag him (her) away from watching a television programme. Perhaps these few words exchanged will be the first steps in getting well again. "When can I see you? This evening?" I always try to go as soon as is convenient.

At this stage I know nothing about the family so I prepare to enter a home which may be either a palace or something less grand. We all take a mental note of what a visitor wears and we tend to react to the clothes worn. Just think of the effect of the doctor's white coverall and you will know what I mean. My clothes therefore must be easy, bland and must conform as much as possible with my hosts' style of living. I go to the toilet before the visit so that the forthcoming interview is not interrupted by my discomfort. Mentally, as the door is answered, I try to conform to the pattern of behaviour that is expected. I allow the scene to be set either on a one to one basis in the bedroom with the spouse busy elsewhere, or in the sitting room with the spouse present, perhaps sitting at a distance, possibly talking to a friend, or sitting close to the patient with the two holding hands.

Just think which of these scenes gives me greatest hope. Why should I waste their time and mine if the two of them cannot share this problem in their lives together? I watch for body language in the same way as I am aware of my own body. I do not comment; I say little except to ask how I can help. What I do is to observe, to be aware and to listen with my heart. Normally I am offered a drink but not a meal and that's fine because this first interview is important. Once the scene is set, perhaps we take the phone off the hook and shut the door. It is in a way a confession, starting with the medical details. Names of doctors and medicine float across but mean little to me as this is not my area and they are aware that I have no medical knowledge, only the experience of being on the receiving end of medicine as a patient.

Once we clear the medical details the talk becomes more personal. "How do you think your cancer was caused?" In the majority of cases we discover some possible reasons. This can take time. Usually a minimum of two hours, more likely four hours or even longer. I get to know the family better perhaps than anyone else. Discoveries are made that even the family don't know about. I invite total truth to be shared across the family so that the problems are equally understood by all the members. I listen to the tenses used: "What we *were* going to do" is bad. "What we *will* do" is good and an affirmation of intent.

As the story unfolds, I reflect that here again is my story. I could be hearing my very own story, only the names are changed. The song they sing may be your tune too. Each time is a learning and relearning experience—about my own weaknesses. An example may be "boredom with life", the fact that there is nothing to achieve, that the children of the home have left to seek their independence, that the parents have only themselves and life has become an endless round of negative actions.

The typical day may go like this:

1 Wake up (badly)
2 Dress (casually)
3 Breakfast (on wrong food)
4 Go to work (unwillingly)
5 "Did you see TV/dreadful weather"
6 Work (no interest)
7 Lunch (on wrong food)
8 "What's on TV/weather's getting worse"
9 Work (no interest)
10 Go home (vacantly)
11 Watch TV (eat wrong food)
12 Fall asleep (nobody talked)
13 Go to bed with a list of problems and no love (sex perhaps, but no love)

Perhaps the problem is boredom about work (or boredom without work). Life becomes meaningless. Bad habits start—like smoking. As more and more negative actions invade the life, the quality diminishes. The problems escalate and although they only reside within the mind they begin to take over like aliens from another planet. Despair, distress, divorce, disaster follow fast—as I know to my cost. There seems to be a macabre form of pleasure in how often 'bad luck' looms larger and larger and so cancer manifests itself as a form of wish fulfillment.

I can imagine that you who read what I have just written are saying "All that is nothing like my past"—maybe so. Perhaps you are young and have breast cancer— so why have you got this illness. Have you been on the pill? Have you had affairs of the heart too often? If you are a mother, have you naturally breast fed your children? Has your past life been totally blameless? Haven't you somehow abused yourself sexually? Most cancers are preventable and are found mainly in persons guilty of self abuse. Just know that cancers are less common in disciplined societies —it is for example rare for nuns to have cancer of the neck of the womb, while Mormon groups living in the United States have an unusually low incidence of all cancers.

The counsellor's aims

In my counselling I am seeking the truth for the particular patient and this can be genuinely hidden from view. Perhaps the possible cause of the problem is the contraceptive pill being used too long, perhaps combined with smoking. Perhaps it is hyperactivity in a job, or the loss of or lack of a job, perhaps bad eating habits or lack of exercise or a combination of these. Perhaps the problem is an emotional one over the spouse, family, lover, work and so on. Possibly the demon drink is the problem, or drugs. Whatever the causes are I listen to learn what the tell-tale clues are. The clues may not lie within the personal control of the cancer patient. The husband may have cancer because the wife drinks or shop lifts or is unfaithful. Any combination amounts to suppressed stress and once these causes are known, are totally out in the open, then the counselling has achieved a first important step.

Remember the clues may not lie in the recent past—they can be hidden, their origins going back many years and there may be many different factors at work. Children suffering from cancer may have to look to their parents either before or after their birth. Did mother smoke when she was pregnant? Although we may not find all the causes we might find enough to learn more about our problem and how we are going to deal with it. Learning to say sorry and to forgive is a good start if the messages are honest. Confession is therefore good for the soul if the confessor truly repents. Forgiveness then becomes easy. The slate is wiped clean and life can begin afresh on the firm understanding that a new chapter begins.

Many doctors do not agree with this point of view, seeing cancer as some form of infection, like smallpox, waiting for the miracle vaccine. There is no doubt that medicine is making great progress all the time to improve the 'cure rates'. However, the cancer is imbedded in us for such a long time before proper action is taken that the disease can well have the upper hand. In any event none of us like to change the habits of a lifetime yet that is what the counsellor must advise if true success is to result.

Some common factors

I have seen so many with cancer, talked with them, wept with them, to know that cancer is a cruel disease. It seems only to affect those who genuinely care more for others than themselves. Are you one of this nature? If you are, if you give 110 per cent of yourself in service of family and others, now is the time to re-direct that love to you alone. Allow others to channel their love to you unconditionally. This is the gentle way and it works. Look at me.

Never be invaded and used. You are not guilty for your past mistakes. It was just a learning experience. Unshackle yourself. Do not conform to others but find the freedom of your own will. You are in control of all the love that happens (or does not happen) within and around you. Use that love wisely.

Are You Giving 110 Per Cent Positively?

Well are you? Reading this book and acting on it? Doing is important. Already I have said to you, action now. I mean it. I have nothing to lose. But you have. Do you really want to get better? Many people with cancer are so overwhelmed by the news that they seem totally incapable of doing anything. I know I felt that, as though a cobra had me in his eyes and just swayed hypnotically before me, ready to strike. That overwhelmed feeling did not last long, Rosemary saw to that. Surely there have been times in your life when total disaster has loomed before you. Somehow you made a plan of action and by others' good help you won through.

Know that a feeling of despair is as common as spots with measles. The lonely feeling of being unwanted and unloved overcomes us all from time to time. Perhaps three times in a minute, an hour, a day. A yogi knows how to detach from such involved negativity . Allow the mind to take a pace back and let the thoughts flow in an uncluttered way. The adrenalin which helps us to deal efficiently with the physical problems in life like fighting to get on a bus or jumping out of its way also acts as poison to our immune system when we are not being physical. So sitting still while allowing adrenalin to course through our body while we grieve over our cancer actually feeds or helps the cancer.

You can see that your body needs to work out these attacks of stress. Working out physically, as I have already suggested, may now seem to be really sensible. I don't mind what stage you are at, from bedridden to leading a normal life, you can always work yourself just that bit harder to improve your physical being. Giving 110 per cent to yourself instead of to others is vitally important. "Who is going to get my husband's (wife's) early cup of tea? And meals? Who is going to do the ironing, washing, mow the lawn, etc?" My answer is that if that work is done as a duty rather than in love then the duty must be stopped—let others take over. Instead, start doing things that you really love and enjoy, spoiling yourself while still physically and mentally exercising.

What about a walk in the country with a drawing book and paints. Who cares if you can't draw or paint. We have all got to start sometime. How about now. What about the family. Are they crowding you? Perhaps the older ones could start pulling their weight by contributing to the chores. A rearrangement to your benefit is necessary, to allow you to be wholly in charge within your home and to become 110 per cent you, is what is needed.

Cancer is a time of change. That change must benefit you, and strangely, you will find it benefits the others around you too. One positive action sets in train many others. I have mentioned this before: positive energy generates many positive results in a similar way that negative energy produces more negativity. Suddenly you must be active and do.

How Pets can Help

I read somewhere that as the elderly grow older and become less active they become more and more housebound. Their world shrinks inward all the time, to their home and garden, then to just their home, their room, their bed, themselves and finally nothing. Cancer is a short cut to that *finality* if this is the genuine inner (and perhaps deeply hidden) desire. So cancer and old age have factors in common. In fact it is true to state that we actually choose the length of life we wish to lead. If we are negative in our attitudes and actions we may be old in our twenties. Others are positively young in their eighties.

Honey is our small poodle. She is a loving member of our family. When there is a gap in the relationship between me and my family Honey is there. A small growl and a play with a toy bring a smile to us all and the bad moment is gone. Pets are simple but genuine beings. Rosemary gave me Honey as a present as I was recovering. A pet is no good to a dying man and this was Rosemary's firm affirmation for my future. She did not say anything like that but there is no doubt that that was her underlying message. Thank you dear one.

Dogs need walks so Honey exercises me. Dogs need love and Honey gives that in the way she can. Dogs need care and attention and this is what we share. My children call Honey my child substitute—perhaps this is true. I have already mentioned that one notices in counselling the use of tenses in sentences. Rosemary's present of the dog Honey to me was an action equally as positive as an affirmation of what we 'will' do for the future. Learn to use affirmative tenses in your thoughts, words and actions—'I will' and 'I can' where appropriate.

Look into your own life and needs. Have you an active pet such as a dog? If you have, share your problems, as I have done. If you have no dog, why not think about getting one? If you truly intend to live then getting a dog or a similar pet could be a good physical step forward. Consider again the elderly, slowly allowing themselves to shrink inwards. Just think of the effect of their taking responsibility for a pet. Would they allow the pet to die for lack of heat or lack of food or lack of exercise if they loved them? Think of cancer as a form of premature dying arising out of negative desires. A pet can be part of the resolution to live if you allow your love to expand in that way.

Finding the Rhythm of Life

All matter is subject to the natural laws of rhythm. Tides of the oceans ebb and flow, day follows night, the breath in our bodies, the beat of our hearts, the periodical rhythm of our bodies day by day and month by month, all respond to the rhythm of life. It is within our power to change the rate of some of these rhythms, especially those within our bodies. The rhythms of the universe are the music of life, of love. Climb up a few flights of stairs and your heart will escalate the rate of pumping. Sit still for a time and the rate will return back to a more normal rate. Longer term changes in our body rhythm can be called a kind of 'jet lag'. The physical changes of jet lag also affect our mental workings so that it is unwise to enter into business discussions immediately after you have flown halfway round the world.

Such changes in the natural rhythms of life are well known. Less well known are the imbalances in our daily lives, the small but gradual pieces of wrong living and thinking and doing that build up until we are out of balance. When do we recognise that we are burning ourselves out, that we sleep badly and work badly? The answer lies within each of us. We each have certain strengths to enable us to overcome imbalances but it is the weak who fall first. Cancer or similar degenerative diseases are illnesses of the weakened spirit which is off balance and has lost that rhythm of life, of love.

We have already discussed yoga and its benefits but perhaps you can now understand that cancer patients who become aware of their problems instinctively turn to yoga. This discipline if properly followed helps to open up the body, mind and spirit to a balanced rhythm of life. It is as simple and as profound as that. If you feel that one class of yoga a week will put you right then you are mistaken. It is more, much more than that. Only you can discover your own imbalances and correct them to your natural rhythm and to learn how years of improper living need to be corrected. Don't ask how, just know that it is so. Remember that we are not aware of all the forces that surround us—either we are young and ignorant or we are older and less aware. Here is an example of my being young and unaware. Has something like this ever happened to you?

When I was in my late teens I worked on board tramp steamers as an ordinary seaman. The job did not last long but the memories of those days are still crystal clear. On one occasion our ship was butting its way slowly across the heavy swell of the North Atlantic. I got up early to view the dawn from the bows of the ship. I stood at the very point where the ship cleaved its way through the heavy seas. The wind made my eyes run and I watched the majesty of a truly wonderful dawn. The sun coloured the clouds deep red, slowly brightened to orange and then crack—the first segment of the sun came into view over the horizon. Soon the rays began to radiate towards me. I was cold and hungry for my breakfast but the spell of this natural event held me. I looked down again at the sea, the colour of which was changing from black and white foam to a pale green frothing torrent. Suddenly a rogue wave slapped the vessel and the water sprayed high all around. I felt wet but remained where I was as I thought it was only a rogue wave and there could be no more like that. I had been, if you like, the ship's figurehead for an hour and I decided to wait until the sun was properly risen and breakfast was ready. Almost as soon as I had made up my mind, cold as I was, I quickly learnt of my error. Almost without stopping the seas came pouring high up over the bows. The dry decks were awash with the constant downpour of salt water. My feelings of being in touch and on nodding terms with nature disappeared. I was racked with terror to get off the fo'c'sle as fast as my feet could take me. I scrambled back to my quarters and quickly changed into dry clothes. I was last in the breakfast line, my teeth chattering with cold, and I was grateful for warmth and food.

Several days after this I became aware that the officers would break out in smiles on seeing me—the greenhorn of the crew. Sadly it took a long time for me to learn the true story of my soaking and how I had been shown to be the sucker I was. Unknown to me as I stood in the bows, the alert bridge officer saw me as a spot of sport and wagered that he could force me off the bows without removing his hands from the wheel. Others on the bridge watched as the wheel man requested that the engine room provide some extra revolutions so as to hold the ship's course better. Naturally the increase in speed increased the bow waves—and I was forced to retreat.

Even now I still find it hard to accept this incident as a joke — as everyone else did. The point is that we are all subject to equally strong pressures from all areas of our lives. Try to be aware of the pressures that have caused the cancer within your perfectly normal body and record your findings in your dairy.

Chapter 9

INSPIRATIONS

Do You Truly Intend to Live?

At the start of this book I suggested we dealt with your cancer problem as if you and I were on a journey. In all journeys we need a rest. We need to discover how far we have travelled, how far we have to go, whether we are on the right path. We must replenish, revitalise, as well as rest. Up to now I have provided you with plenty of material for your journey. We have if you like covered the easy part, the valley part, of the journey and now we look upwards.

Upwards are the mountains we will climb together. The obstacles appear formidable and well beyond our strength. You feel fear and deeply wish to turn back to your old ways. You and I sit on a small hillock by the path and here we find out much about each other that we did not discover at the start of our journey. You start to ask me questions like:

Q: "Can I go on?"

A: "Yes".

Q: "What makes you certain?"

A: "What makes you (uncertain) think you can turn your face against what lies ahead? You will be letting yourself down, as well as your family, friends, doctors, nurses and me. We have spent our time and energy to get you this far. Why turn back now? Why give in to negativity? Why lose the battle before it has tested you?"

Q: "Colin, I will go on provided you allow me the option to change my mind at any time."

A: "Of course. You are in control. You alone are in charge of your future. All I am inviting you to do is to accept the challenge of the mountain. To know that others do succeed and there is every reason why you can succeed as well."

The will to succeed

You should now feel within you a surge of confidence that the mountains of doubt can be overcome with the help of those around you who love you. Success is 10 per cent inspiration, 90 per cent perspiration. Think 'success' every moment by your every action. Know that your surgery scars are battle scars. Your medication is the test of yourself, tests which are your local victories. Each time you visit your hospital they are giving you the essential supplies that a soldier requires in battle.

Your journey is therefore made as an advancing soldier against a retreating enemy who is taking to the mountains to stage his final defence. You feel that your cause is right. You truly intend to live and with your strength recovered you wish to be on your journey. Know now that your cause is right and that you are on your way. "Just a moment", I caution. "Just make sure you know your objectives—and your battle cry!" "My objectives are clear, Colin", you answer. "To rid my body and mind of all cancerous aspects that have invaded me. To achieve these objectives I will employ totally the skills of the doctors and nurses in whom I place my faith. In addition I will employ all the complementary treatments that are available to me and which I feel will assist me and not conflict with my medication. Finally I will bring myself to a state of personal readiness so my sheer positiveness will overwhelm everyone, both the enemy and my friends. I know it is all up to me and my inner convictions."

Arming for the fight

"Colin, I see that what I have been told by you up to now is really just a list of ingredients. I have to select those that are right for me, depending on my health and determination to win. I must make my own menu as each of us is unique. What may be good for me may not be good for you. Yes, Colin, I understand I am in charge. I am refreshed, I want to get on. I am stripping myself of all unnecessary burdens in order to climb these mountains—and this means a differently equipped soldier to the trainee soldier newly conscripted and burdened with untried, untested weapons. But Colin, what is the battle cry?

"The battle cry is the one word which I feel sums up this book: — PURIFICATION".

Knowing in your imagination that you are an experienced soldier you take up only that equipment which will help you in the next part of your journey. You feel inspired and are ready and eager to be off. You feel as though you are the white knight, wholly immune within, confidently armed without. With this attitude of confidence in your very being there is no doubt that you truly intend to live. The passive acceptances, the doubts, the rubbish of your former self have been left by the wayside. What I have advised and lovingly shared with you has ignited a flame of desire such as you have never previously experienced. You the ordinary person in the valley becomes the extra-ordinary properly inspired 'Joan of Arc' of the mountains beyond the valley.

Making your choice

In counselling work I can see those who suddenly know for the first time what has to be done, the eyes are suddenly opened and the change is magic. The knowing is all important. Conversely there are others, young in body, torn in mental conflict to whom I have asked that essentially fundamental question "Do you truly intend to live?" They have divided loyalties between home, parents, comfort, security or alternatively a fresh place to live, a lover, no comfort, no security. Which do they choose? If they lean more towards home, then intense pressure is imposed by the lover. However, if the lover is more attractive then the parents or family may cling instead of letting go. Hopefully such a cancer patient can find a true resolution to this problem and become a white knight. Unfortunately this is not always the case and the red knight (cancer) wins.

Inspirations for Children with Cancer

Young children with cancer are only young persons with stresses similar to adults. Here one should look more and more towards the parents for the cause of the cancer. Has the child been rejected or fought over by the parents? Is the home or school environment bad? Is the child bullied or torn emotionally in some other way? A husband and wife may be locked in an endless war and at each others throats. They are the cause but the child suffers by being unable to live a healthy life in such an acidly cancerous place even although it is called home.

In such situations the cancer patient is uninspired, has not got the will or inner fire to live. The seed of their own self destruction is sown and this seed grows into reality and is granted in death. Naturally the patient and the causative agents (the parents) need to recognise this problem. All must agree to do something about it and then to carry it out. The cross of life is too heavy and has to be cast aside so that in an unburdened way the mountains of doubt can be climbed and conquered.

In practical terms it means a change of ways for the child and the parents. This can mean separation so the decisions have to be fairly made and honestly kept. Love for the cancer patient may mean emotional sacrifices to those involved.

Belief is Greater Than All Medicine

So here we are leaving our resting place behind. You as the white knight for once take the lead. No more do you tag behind. No more are your questions asked with head hung low. Confident in your decisions and with a firm belief in the correctness of your aims you climb the foothills of the mountains. Hardly a backward glance at me your guide. Your zeal is such that you increase your pace as the going gets harder.

Climbing mountains is an art. The art is not in rushing

forward but in learning by watching a true mountaineer. Such an expert is properly prepared and sets off at a steady firm pace. The pace is set by the size of the mountain ahead and the known strength of the expert. This belief in conquering mountains is the quality I wish to discover in those who start to take control of their cancer. It is a quality that is found in matters we have discussed such as yoga, music, relaxation, healing and so on. The quality is in the firmness, truth and slow rhythmical strength of the belief in getting well in spite of all barriers. It is a magical quality that has to be worked for in order to attain it and sheer dedication is needed.

Belief in yourself

As I write this book I endeavour to instil in my (and your) very being once again that the belief is greater than all medicine. To describe the indescribable is impossible—like trying to define infinity. Yet I need to nurture my belief that what I am doing is right for me. I am no superman, far from it. I am too human, but I need constantly to draw from within affirmations for the rightness of my actions and attitudes. Naturally there are those who disagree and their attitudes may be right for themselves. Belief is simple and personal. If you want to find belief then it is through the action of your own self discovery. There are for example many therapies giving different approaches to healing. If your attitudes (as mine were initially) are that such therapies in complementing conventional medicine will not work for you, then this 'disbelief' becomes your 'belief'. It is your burden, your attitude. Certainly if your views are that all available therapies won't work, then they won't. Your inner wish is fully and wholly granted. Your resistance blocks you from climbing your mountain by one path. You will have to find another way up.

However, just suppose you are prepared to consider placing yourself in the hands of a local therapist and allowing them to assist your healing then your scepticism may be a burden you cast off. This opening of your awareness to the healing channels available to you will only work if you allow an inner co-operation to flow. Unblocking your scepticism is difficult but when you are confronted with a life-threatening illness, I for one, was not prepared nor able to stand in the way of any therapy I or my Rosemary felt might help me. I therefore allowed my belief to enfold such matters as natural remedies, homoeopathy, spiritual healing and prayer. As my belief expanded so my desire to live improved. I looked out for further therapies which I could test and use, or reject as not being for me. The rejection could be that I did not accept the person involved or the therapy suggested. If they seemed suitable and I accepted the possible value of the therapy, then my belief played its part in that therapy. This is part of your way forward in climbing your mountain. It is a committed inner belief and that will be your strength.

Finding the true self

You will find a help in your search for the way upwards to good health in quiet meditation. Somehow the quietening of the body and the mind puts you in tune with your true self. You slowly draw strength from within and become re-energised. Who has not seen this in others facing impossible odds? Somehow they seem to surmount the ordeal both stronger and wiser. Certainly those who have survived cancer are committed persons. They have run long distances, climbed mountains and continue to do such incredible feats. Just know that in your inner silence you too can find the peace and stillness of your self from which natural area will grow the seeds of belief and inner conviction (a determination of what is right for *you*) which will allow you to set a firm pace. Some might say that what you have permitted in allowing these seeds of belief to grow is for the voice of God to be heard.

Religions

I would not interfere / with any creed of yours
Or want to appear / that I have all the cures
There is so much to know / so many things are true . . .
The way my feet must go / may not be best for you
And so I give this spark / of what is light to me

To guide you through the dark / but not tell you what to see

— *Anon*

I approach this subject with great care. Almost at once I am aware that I intrude on something that is totally fundamental to you the reader. Even if you don't practise any religion, you will possibly still have strong views on the subject of religion. In many places such as clubs there are rules that religion, politics and sex are subjects not to be discussed.

Cancer is a 'dis-ease'—you are not at ease. Religions provide codes of beliefs about both the supernatural and the natural to ease the spirit and the real needs of man. I admit to being a 'non-attending' practising Church of England Protestant. I am 'non-attending' because in the past attendance has never provided me with the sincere satisfaction I feel I need. Perhaps I should look to other religions. But do they provide what we or I am seeking?

What exactly do we seek from religion? Well, we wish to be motivated to lead a better life in all ways. This includes health. At one time it used to be the parish priest who provided help be it spiritual or physical. The priest would have been a healer and would have heard your confessions. Somehow along our history there has been parting of the ways. The healing aspect has fallen into the hands of the doctors, whereas the spiritual aspects have become split into a multitude of religions each proclaiming its own rightness. Ordinary mortals are confused. We are simple people who do not wish to be involved in the time-wasting arguments of dogmas. We do not wish to fight each other for the sake of our masters. We seek and need help on a total personal level. How do we get in touch with God? How can we pray for help? I am ill in body, mind and spirit; I need comfort, care, compassion. As the Church appears to fail to meet or understand the needs of the person it becomes obvious that the positive aspects religions can offer diminish and negative aspects of non-religious behaviour increase bringing with it the increase in cancers, AIDS, and similar conditions.

Yes, this is a generalisation, and yes, I know of priests who serve their flock faithfully providing comforts on all levels. However, do you not agree that the proper thrust of the Churches and religions is to meet the physical, mental as well as the spiritual needs of the modern person, and this is not happening. More and more people are turning away because it does not attract. People look to me for healing and in the cause of love I offer what I can and pray that their needs are fulfilled. Yet I am angry that our so-called 'people of religion' do not boldly step into the hospitals, hospices and homes and offer healing as Christ and other great persons have done. Perhaps I see it all in simple terms but doctors and priests should draw together in an effort to undo the cancerous splitting and subdividing that has happened down the centuries. There should be unity within all religion and medicine so that they become one.

The comfort of belief

How do you feel about religion? Does it give you spiritual comfort? If so, then use the strength of your faith and learn to pray for guidance for an improvement in your health. When I think of prayer I am reminded of the story of the soldier who was returning from leave and going back to the front line. On the transport there were many soldiers who had yet to hear a gun fired in anger. Their group fun and jollity spilled over into ribald ridicule of the soldier kneeling by his bunk. The soldier completed his prayers and stood up to confront his comrades. "When you have been into the fire of battle, when you have seen death in the face and your comrades are no more, then you will learn to pray", he said.

The attitude of the soldier with experience touched the spirit of the others who quietly began to follow his example of prayer. Thus is it so with cancer; it is just another battle. It is said that the wounded on the battle field in crying for help, cry for their mothers or God. They do not normally cry for their spouse, or children. At such times the truth of the spirit pervades the wounded warrior. Cancer is a similar battle ground and spiritual strength should be sought in prayer. If your religion, and more importantly your local religious leader, can give you this strength then do not hesitate to ask. That leader may actually learn from you as you learn from him. My meditation includes a prayer at the start; the prayer involves my family and friends that collectively we will always assist each other at times of need and that we may be guided to do the right thing for each other. I find the following prayer a great comfort and joy in writing this book for you.

Lord make me an instrument of your peace
Where there is hatred, let me sow love
Where there is injury, pardon
Where there is doubt, faith
Where there is darkness, light
Where there is despair, hope
Where there is sadness, joy

Divine master, grant that I may not so much seek
To be consoled as to console
To be understood as to understand
To be loved as to love
For it is in giving that we receive
It is in pardoning that we are pardoned
And in dying that we are born to eternal life

The Breath of the Spirit

Earlier in the book I pointed out how important the breath was. Yes I know we all breathe and it is the most important function of our body. I suggested that you would be wise to learn how to breathe properly. A good yoga teacher would assist you, and that teacher would tell you that through breath you took in an energy called *prana*. Prana is an essential quality of life; it is most in a healthy person and least in a dying person. It exists in all life, plant as well as animal. In some way it can be measured by Kirlian photography. This is a simple matter of putting a photo sensitive paper into a special machine and placing a part of our body such as the hand on it. Switching on the machine produces an outline of the hand on the photo sensitive paper. The paper will also show in detail flares of energy escaping from our fingers similar to flares escaping from the sun. These flares are pranic energy and the bigger and more dense they are the greater is the discharge. An experienced healer would record large flares and a dying person a few small flares. There is still much research to be done on this subject but already some interesting discoveries are being made. It is if you like a physical proof of our auric spirit. It is able to detect illness and types of disease by absences of energy.

By placing food on a Kirlian machine you can measure the amount of pranic energy that the food contains. If you repeat the measurement a day later the energy will be less, showing that fresh food is better for us and more vital than stale food. Place a leaf on the machine and again the energy pattern will appear. The outline of the leaf will be clear. Now tear away a segment of leaf, say a quarter, and throw the quarter away. Now place the three-quarter segment of the leaf on the machine and amazingly the machine will photograph what is not there. The complete outline will be visible although the torn-away section will be slightly less prominent.

How can a machine actually photograph something that is not there? It is as if the spirit of life (prana) of the leaf remains for a time intact in spite of the physical loss. Similarly, on losing a leg, the patient experiences the need to scratch the leg which is no longer there. As science unfolds the mysteries of nature we should be prepared to open our awareness to ideas and facts which the majority may still feel are fictions. Why do we not believe in miracles, of matters not scientifically proven? Can you not extend the areas of your understanding to take in the mysteries that exist just around the corner. I don't know how a television works but I do know that if I have a set and electric power then coloured pictures will appear on one side of the set. Is that not a miracle that we accept without scientific proof? Therefore in your cancer problem can you accept the breath of the spirit to help you get better?

Chapter 10

TRANSFORMATIONS

Death; Your Rights

Death is a parting and you should consider this honestly within yourself and then discuss it openly with your family. To hide a problem is a burden which you should not have to impose on yourself. Children should also be told and prepared for death in a kind way so that this caring attitude can bring a loving response from them. In this way they can help and feel part of the family in trouble and they will not feel left out in the event of death.

Death of part of the body

Cancer operations always involve an element of risk—all operative procedures on the body do. Nevertheless you must believe in and be comforted by the skill (generally high) of surgeons, doctors and of course nurses. Operations are normally performed only when there is a justifiable element of success. The surgical removal of part of the body—that is the part that has cancer tissue—is like a death of part of yourself. An internal operation will result in some change in the body functions for the future. It is up to you to see that the care by doctors is continued by yourself afterwards even if you think it is not necessarily your problem. Be comforted to know that given the right care, our bodies can still function excellently with various parts removed.

Life post-operatively

After an operation, the patient may have to alter their way of life in some way and that is why I have indicated that the problem of care lies in the patient's hands when the doctors have done their duty. So many people I see seem to feel that their body is the sole concern of the doctor. They seem to disassociate their bodies from themselves. "Colin, I will see what the doctors suggest next time I go", you say. "Yes, but what do *you* feel and think should be done?", I reply. "Oh, Colin, I don't know; it is not up to me, is it?" 'Well, yes it is. Don't divorce yourself from the problem. Be in there and offer what you know about yourself. The doctors like to have all the clues that it is possible to give them. Don't hide a lump or some other known physical symptom from them'.

In my own case, with part of my stomach removed, people say "But Colin, how can you eat?" Quite well thank you, provided I am careful to eat little and often. Naturally I am examined at intervals and sometimes I have a worry so I report my concern promptly to my doctor rather than wait for the next appointment. So part of my body has died and gone forever but what remains adjusts and with my care of my inner disability plus the regular confirmation from my doctors, we seem to be making good progress as a team. That is how it should be.

The operation I had was an internal one; the scars are hardly visible. An 'external' operation with visible results brings the added problem of the mental anguish for the patient and also those nearest in love to the patient. The physical removal of the breasts or sexual organs in particular can cause bereavement in a relationship. It is an important problem which must be considered carefully by both doctors, patient and family. It is necessary that a caring attitude is taken so that the shock is minimised. Again, as in death which I mentioned earlier, loving discussion is an essential and necessary part of the preparation. The loss of, for example, a breast is a sexual bereavement—it does not however mean the loss of a sexual relationship. Hopefully, strength and understanding by all concerned can overcome the understandable initial fears.

Death of the whole of the body

This leads me to the death of the whole body rather than the loss of a part or parts. Naturally whether it is loss of part or loss of the

119

whole, grief is involved. And to a greater or lesser extent grief is involved to all those who love you. You may have been emotionally involved in the death of a loved one in the past so you know the feelings that are involved here, the intensity of bereavement and length of time it lasts. 'I shall never get over that loss', you might think. Certainly bereavement involves change and it may well be that this grief is a cause of your cancer. Unsupported grief is a step towards a person's own cancerous state. Prolonged bereavement is many steps down this path. Consider my problem and note that I could not handle my own sorrow about my parents in an appropriate way.

With hindsight I now see that those old ghosts still haunted me. Do you not agree that such matters lay the foundations for cancer to occur? When I was eleven the liner I was aboard was torpedoed in a North Atlantic gale. I spent twenty hours in a lifeboat watching most of the other passengers drowning or dying of exposure. At the time of my rescue I was praised for my bravery but frankly I wanted to grieve and I needed tears and compassion. Brave boys don't cry so I stoically held back what I needed to vent in the way of my feelings.

My own emotional 'history'

My father died of leukaemia when I was in my early thirties. That grief I could handle because his illness had been discussed along with the chances of his survival or death. In a way I was properly prepared, and when his death came, I was sad but comforted by my family. However, my mother did not have the comfort she needed and she committed suicide by taking an overdose a few hours later. It was I who discovered her body in bed when I went into her bedroom with her usual early morning tea. My mother had solved her problem but had left a deep emotional scar on the family. It has taken me weeks of agony to write these words. They are torn from my heart, covered in tears. Emotionally I am drained every time the matter is raised. Yet for my own good these words had to be written and shared with you so that you know you are not alone. We all have historical ghosts.

The point I wish to share with you is that these events

happened roughly 50 years and 25 years ago respectively. The agony of them lingers on, however, because I was not helped through my grief in the way I now feel to be important. You will find a further expansion of this topic in the details of books by Elisabeth Kübler-Ross at the end of this book. We all need help and counselling from those outside the family circle who can show care, compassion and competence. Yet grief is only a mental problem, or is it? Can you not see that as a result of this mental anguish your body systems firmly shut down so that the bereaved person is inwardly calling for a similar fate to occur? "Life is not worth living; what shall I do; I can't sleep in spite of the pills the doctor has given me"—these are the expressions we use. Anger and despair are what govern the bereaved person.

The trauma often gets worse. Offers of help from family and friends are listened to and ignored. There seems to be no resolution. Every moment is beautiful agony and this negativity radiates outwards to upset those around. Then the bereaved feel they are truly and absolutely deserted and the emotional state of health gets worse and worse. Those with cancer may be concerned about their own death. But if what I say has any influence on you then you may feel you ought to do more to stay alive and to spare your family the bereavement problem that will follow. Bereavement as I describe it in my own case can lie within the self for many years. It is your own atomic explosion, causing a gradual erosion of your inner defence, your immune system, over the years through worry and fears about day to day matters so that you react wholly in excess of the normal reaction to the stresses of life. The atomic bombs which fell on Japan in 1945 are still causing higher than normal rates of cancer more than 40 years later. The problems of the human body and the human race are similar except in scale.

Discussing death

We are all, frankly, unwilling, unprepared and fearful of death. It is a wise patient who brings up the subject and the future for his or her family to discuss and it is a sensible family who are prepared to listen and contribute usefully to the discussion. This can ease the minds of all and once discussed the subject can be placed to one side while all efforts are made to get well again. There are those who 'know' death is not far away and who are afraid. Here true love comes forth in allowing the last moments to be a release of those last wishes and thoughts. It would seem sensible to draw up a code of conduct: who is to be there and who is not. In the last moments, as the senses slowly withdraw, it is important to know that the brain can still function after the breath has gone. In those last moments therefore we should continue in affirmations of our love and release so that in the patient's dying experience there is the hearing of their loved ones' messages.

Many people have experienced what is called a 'near death' experience. The similarity and number of such happenings can only lead one to believe that there is a welcome on the far side of death. The spirit therefore moves on leaving the body behind in the same way that the butterfly escapes from its chrysalis, or the light flows on from an electric lamp into infinity long after the lamp goes out. 'Near death' experience literally means that people have begun the actual death event but that the process has reversed or been reversed for some reason. All have felt incredible waves of welcome, of light at the end of a tunnel, and of a desire to move towards the light. It is if you like a reverse of the birth experience. There is definitely a feeling of resentment if the death process is reversed and life is reawakened in the person. It seems as if it is a sad letdown! Treat death as a blessed release. When I saw my mother's body it was not my mother—and she as the human spirit she was had definitely gone. The object of my affection as my mother was no longer in that room. Since that time my inner grief still yearns over this loss and maybe I have made the parting difficult because I have been unable to 'let go'. This feeling is called having 'unfinished business'. Have you any unfinished business?

Doctors and nurses can assist in the comfort of the dying person with the help of drugs. Therefore the fear of death should not be uppermost but rather a feeling of relief from illness and the freedom of the spirit. We should not selfishly wish for prolonged life if death is a natural release. Having experienced the miracle of birth with the birth of my children and the awareness that after birth there is another soul spirit in the room I feel that we should consider death as being the exact opposite. The cyclical rhythm of life moves on and we cannot struggle against the changes that are constantly with us. If you have a priest to counsel you on this matter so that you are able to talk openly and happily on this subject then you should do so earlier rather than later. This person can offer you solace and comfort in addition to prayers. Hopefully they may be able to advise you on more practical matters of the body and mind in addition to caring for your spiritual needs.

Perhaps I have opened up channels of discussion for you and those nearest to you. Now put the problem away as it has been dealt with in the spirit of love. At the beginning of Chapter 9 we had a rest and discussion and at the end we talked about problems dealt with promptly and firmly and without regrets. Have you been able to do this? If you have then this clears your mind and reveals your proper mental attitude to your cancer by leaving no stone unturned. Now step on upwards.

Life One Step At a Time

Each day in your life is a step on your path. Each step is a knowing of self improvement or not. At the same time, each day you must factually examine yourself. You must overcome the fear shock waves to which we as cancer patients are all subjected and record your findings of your body and your inner mental state. This self appraisal and reappraisal is important. Are you worse or better? Is this because of the treatment received? Is the cancer receding or advancing? You must muster your inner strengths and reserves and note your findings in your diary. What are your plans for today? How can you minute-by-minute ensure that you are being purified by what you eat, drink, think, believe? What new plans have you to ensure that you are not just sitting on your hands either physically or mentally? Recognise the cancerous symptom of wanting to throw in the towel, to give up. Know that large armies not properly motivated can be allowed to surrender to small invasive forces. Your body may be like that large army; it may have got lazy in its ways. Nature looks kindly on a body that is used properly, efficiently, in the way it was conceived. Where did you go wrong and what are you doing to correct the imbalance within you?

Even if what you do is judged 'wrong' by the experts, the experts do not have cancer and you do! Know that the 'doing' is essential. Nothing is useless. Actively 'doing' and believing one hundred per cent is what is required. "OK, Colin, I have got the message", you say. "Really I am being exceptionally positive and everybody is pleased with my progress. I understand what you wrote earlier about striding up my mountain. These are my problems, to be tackled by me. Yes I have some support in various ways, but I must be the white knight climbing that mountain in order to utterly destroy all that cancerous negativity that builds up within me".

A call to arms

Right! Do you feel inspired like a soldier responding to the beat of the drum. Do you feel a freedom of action and a joy of purpose. Can you throw off the shackles of the death bed, bed pan, etc. Can you use the treatments as weapons to throw back the invasion rather than allow them to hasten your decline. Draw on your courage and become inspired to show that in spite of everything you will succeed. With a coming to terms with this new attitude, your zeal for life, carefully increasing with each stride, will give you the victory you seek. Your body will respond to the mental positiveness I am instilling into your inner self. No longer are you considering the downside of cancer, we have even discussed death and know of that matter. Rather we are wholly committed to life and the qualities of life that you have taken for granted in the past.

You must ignore critics and 'downers'. You are rewriting the script of your life and you have become the central character. Your family and friends are now helping you rather than the other way around and no longer do you feel guilty. In fact suddenly you are enjoying a new quality of life. You feel strong in yourself and have a glorious carefree sense of freedom from former shackles. Recognise that your confidence can easily be eroded in the twinkling of an eye or as a result of a chance rotten remark so it is essential to be aware that the new positive you has to retain this quality and radiance always.

As the fears begin to recede and your joy breaks through you will find that your inner mental disciplines of meditation and visualisation are really working. At that stage doctors will become cautiously pleased at your progress, perhaps suggesting that you shouldn't rush too fast. You feel you have nothing to lose; you have stared death in the face and have not elected to die just yet thank you. At this stage cancer patients feel an urge to celebrate, to spend some money, to go to the opera, do something they have never done before. Why not! Some do silly things, only those things are sensible to them: dress up as a clown, release balloons, hug strangers in hospital, so that other people can share their feelings of happiness. This book, if you like, is about my own controlled joy of being. I don't care about anything except to convey to you, my friend, of my ecstasy. Like battle veterans at a reunion, the past is gone only the memories are there, both sad and good, but now I am alive and well. Follow your own route and come and join me at the top of the mountain.

Life a New Direction

We are told that you do not get cured of cancer. The best we are advised is that if you survive free of cancerous symptoms for five years then it is reasonably certain that there will not be a recurrence. A person such as you may ask but what is life like after cancer; it is worth living? You may feel from all that I have written that the best you can expect is a half life as a half person in which no enjoyment can be found. Naturally I can speak only for myself and for those whom I have met who have passed this important milestone. I can honestly say that I am glad I had cancer. My life is better and more fulfilling than it was before. It has been a powerful lesson and not one I would like to repeat. I enjoy my life in my new direction compared to the life I had before having cancer. My answer is similar to others who have been through the experience: we have all learnt valuable lessons and provided we don't forget them, then we shall grow in all ways in the future.

What have I learnt? Well, I am thankful for life and for the skill and dedication of all those who have helped me. I realise in the past that I tried too hard to attain targets and now I see that in simply allowing the natural spirit and energy of myself to evolve I can achieve much more than ever before. Really, I suppose, I hated myself for being unable to achieve, whereas it is only through a loving approach that you can excel. Now I say to myself: "Just how stupid could I have been?"

I see these same stupid attitudes in others, trying to run too hard on life's rim. Presumably they too are at risk of corroding their inner selves into cancer and then having to find their own way through like me. But will they have the good fortune, luck and sheer determination of spirit to come out the other side as a newly changed person? You are going to be OK aren't you? Your inner belief will see to that.

Frankly, as civilization grows, so we enjoy its benefits and start moving into the fast lane of life. You can allow this to happen for a time, but then nature starts taking a hand and the *karma* (or the lesson) and punishment is handed out. It sounds so obvious and so it is. We all play with fire in our individual ways. What I write is no more than good sense to me—good sense that has been discovered the hard way. I know this now, but actually I knew it before: the difference can be summed up as follows: —

You are not taught anything;
Already you know everything;
Only you don't know you know;
Until something —
unshackles the knowledge.

Chapter 11

RELAXATIONS

Letting Go

We are approaching the end of the book. We will have to part and go our different ways soon. Before we part can I try to instil into your very being the importance of change by improving the health essence of your life? I have written about matters that proved good for me, and still do, but they might not be acceptable to you. The importance is in the 'doing' of whatever it is for your own self health improvement. You must motivate yourself to take charge of your well being and not leave the overall responsibility to others.

'Doing' does not actually mean actively moving to or working from place A to place B. Rather it can be the opposite, of just being where you are at place A or place B and letting go. My life involves constantly moving from A to B and back again; this is called commuting. Whilst at B I am under pressure to complete matters of business quickly and effectively or suffer the stresses of others. This means stress on me, on those who work with me, from the highest to the lowest. Am I in control of me?

Is your life like that? Are others taking over control of you so that you are no longer the special personal master of all your space? Are you becoming a slave to others, where your individual thoughts and actions become less and your obedience to rules made by others for others becomes more? Are you an airline traffic controller, pilot or stewardess, housewife, business executive or doctor—any occupation where you can see you are losing your self, your own freedom and health? If your name is called is your reaction within "what have I done wrong?" And with a startled flow of adrenalin scouring through your body systems are you nervous, easily angered but only show the anger in the face and not in full physical reaction? Are you suppressing stress but later turn on others which afterwards you regret? Do you easily lose things and spend time hunting for them, angry with everybody and anything as long as it is not you. Do you find it difficult even to do simple everyday tasks without irritation? Do you hate the weather? Life? Yourself?

Yes?

The stress response habit

When the mind fights itself, the right part of the brain against the left part, we are left in a weakened state, confused. Our brain patterns become distorted, the body is full of unnecessary hormones trying to stimulate but not succeeding. The toxins in the body increase over the years and physical activity, which could help eliminate these poisons, reduces through the passage of time. This is understandable and affects us all to a certain degree. Why all this mental running, running, running? Let's give the body a treat and gently 'push away' all those guilty ghosts of the past and the hyperactivity of the present, eliminating the possible future problems. Let us try to be in the present, calm, controlled, relaxed and letting go of all that stuff.

Allow nothing to distract you, become the calm eye in the middle of the storm around you and maintain that calmness. Just look at how you are reading these words. Are you tense? Just relax. Work around your body carefully, easing out those limbs, uncrossing those legs. Sit up straight and watch your breathing. Take slower, easier breaths, hold each breath for a little longer and exhale slowly. Already your active brain patterns will have started to slow down following my suggestion, sown as a seed in your brain. Watch how your brain reacts in rhythm with your body, one now responding to the other. As your body starts to let go so your brain guides. "This is nice, let's have more". So your body eases again and in turn your brain calms down returning to memory some of those problems that were uppermost in your mind.

Relaxation is an art. Some may find it in watching television.

Have you considered how actively your brain is actually working in watching television? Your eyes receive the message in pictures, your ears the story in words. The input to the brain is large and all is carefully stored away for future recall. How often have you found that in watching a film you have previously seen you can actually recall the entire story and perhaps even the next lines of the actors. So this type of watching television is not letting go, it is the opposite. Are there other ways in which we can delude ourselves that we are relaxing? How about gardening or golf or holidays? Well certainly a change from your normal life routine is very welcome and enjoyable but how easily do you allow yourself to relax? The garden needs constant attention. Leave it a week and say hello to the weeds. The golf is enjoyable until you lose your grip slightly and then things can go from bad to worse. A holiday is fun but there is the organising, the cost, packing, unpacking, travel, different and less satisfactory accommodation, different food and so on. Well yes, there are enjoyable parts in holidays, in anything, but the downside is always there as well so that you may perceive things in a negative attitude of mind.

Finding the calm state within

So let us go back again to the calm eye in the middle of the storm. Let us learn how the two parts of our brain act and react one to the other so that you can say 'I have changed my mind'. Have you changed for the better or for the worst? Who ultimately is in control of you? This interaction within the mind is worrying so it is exhausting and we cry 'help' in some way when we reach an overload. "If you say that once again I'll . . ." Could you really say and do that to someone you know and love? Perhaps an idle threat—or an acute call of agony and despair. You will perhaps realise that meditation properly taught can bring you to a state of quiet mind control whenever you need it. Meditation is practised in many ways but the principle is to reduce the brain wave patterns to an acceptable state of calmness in which state you may commence quietly to meditate. Your body calms, your mind calms and there you are—in peaceful stillness. All is peace within and the healing can commence.

Those who may not understand this natural state of the body need only to think of the time when they wake up in the morning. It is not a work day and so you have woken without an alarm call. There is peace and quiet and your brain is hardly active, just quietly reporting on what is happening . . . "nothing much: a bird is singing, the sun's shining, I am warm, I can't feel my legs, I feel a bit spaced out, where am I—oh, yes, I am at home in my bed, I don't have to get up, I just want to be me, as I am now, relaxed . . ." In that dreamy, half waking, half sleeping state, we are touching that part of our existence about which we know so little—yet it is so enjoyable. Allowing this part conscious, part unconscious effect, tunes you in to meditation. It also tunes you in to your spiritual self so that it becomes a voice of self-discovery, or self learning and self loving.

In finding this spiritual quality you can become more positive in your attitudes because you start to know instead of doubt. As mental stresses reduce so does bodily health improve. Body and mind work once again in harmony by allowing the inner spiritual wisdom to be heard. You are no longer frightened, you are letting go and allowing a surge of fresh energy and life force to go to every part of you. You start looking younger and better. I was asked "Are you in love!" That is exactly it. Don't we all know that perfect state of love? The world is good and we could skip to the songs within us.

The beneficial effects of a calm outlook

Patients with AIDS now use the techniques of mind settling and body calming that I describe in this book. Their defence system, the immune system, is totally collapsed whereas a cancer patient has lost only a part of their defence system. The essential need is to repair these defects in our defences. Anxiety, despair and worry are all allies of cancer growth. They knock away the defences and cancer invades further and faster. Looking at my family's medical reference book, now four years old, I find that almost every possible illness and medical condition is listed. The book also includes information on healthy eating, keep fit, aerobics and yoga. These pages total 33 pages in all—roughly five per cent of the book. This shows a growing awareness that each of us must take proper care of ourselves on a regular basis. It is also interesting to note that there is no reference to AIDS, showing that even four years ago it did not rate a mention. Now it may be a possible world-threatening disease within as short a time as 10 years.

Yoga in all its aspects deals with the health of the body, mind and spirit. It teaches us that you cannot deal with body alone or mind alone or spirit alone. This trinity is essentially inter-related in the way I have described in Chapter 00. A typical yoga class starts with relaxation. Walking into a yoga class is the same as entering the calm eye of the storm. All the customary hyperactivity of life is left behind as yoga students stretch out on the floor in the corpse pose. Each body is totally relaxed, arms and legs away from the body, eyes are closed. The teacher guides students to remove day to day thoughts from the front of their minds and to still their brains—and gradually an all-pervading and calm atmosphere is enjoyably encountered. The strength of this spiritual atmosphere is most soothing—just like that early morning waking state where you don't have to move. In a yoga class you are guided by the teacher and because of the number of students and the joint commitment to the class and what goes on there, the value of a class relaxation is infinitely more beneficial than when done on one's own. There are if you like unwritten rules of discipline and awareness which the whole class willingly and eagerly observe. The class proceeds in this same state of tranquility to do either physical or mental work. You note that while you are moving into a physical posture the calmness and slowness allows your body to move further, the muscles allowing the movement to flow to the fullest extent. During normal movements, muscles move in opposite directions—one set to contract, one set to extend. In slow yogic movement we 'talk' to these muscles, allowing a further extension than would be used in normal activity. This provides youthful flexibility.

The grace of these movements is like ballet and yet within the grasp of all of us. As the movement is performed so the mind is totally involved—it must be in order to harmonise the whole self. No other mental problem can intrude on your yoga. You are in class for your space alone. No longer are you at the beck and call of others, family or friend. For just a short time you enjoy your own self in its stillness and allow the body to repair itself without stress. Yoga therefore is a healing discipline and as natural a function as yawning and stretching when you get out of bed. As you enhance your practice you become aware of the spiritual wholeness. Nothing in natural yoga involves any particular religion or politics, just the recognition of the ultimate reality and the brotherhood of our fellow persons. We are all one.

Arising out of this yogic practice of relaxation comes a whole fresh way of viewing your life. You take what you learn into your life so that everyday tasks are dealt with by you in a different attitude of mind. This extends even to watching television. No longer do you let the pictures and the noise pass over you in an endless wash of useless stuff. You watch what you want then turn it off. Afterwards you talk to your family or do other tasks which need to be done. Your gardening, golf or holidays are gently planned in your mind and enjoyed in this same relaxed state of mind. "Colin", you say, "when I garden I just lose myself. I could be there for an hour or a day—and I become totally in tune with nature". The same with golf "Colin I just don't know how the time goes by. It is a totally enjoyable experience. At one time I began to play badly but then I remembered to relax. I allowed my mind not to interfere with my play; I experienced a feeling that I was watching myself play from a distance. Without my own conscious interference I could observe my play come back to normal and as I continued it became better, better in fact than I have ever played."

Holidays too now become a relaxed form of living, right from the initial conception. In fact you hardly wish to go at all as the anticipation itself is so good. In this relaxed state of mind you can perform any and all tasks of life. By allowing your mind to step back, you can achieve more. A good example of this is long distance running. A novice runner can be defeated before the start of a race just by thinking of the distance they have to run. A good runner knows of barriers that he will encounter as the will and energy start to evaporate after say two thirds the distance. A good relaxed runner will especially atune the mind by allowing a conservation of body energy and a diminution of mind activity.

The art is not to let the mind say to the self that the run is impossible. Instead your run is conducted in that controlled waking dream state described earlier. Your body performs and your mind is quietly detached. Your life should also be led in that pure stress-free and relaxed state of letting go.

Your central question to yourself

I often ask some cancer patients "Do you feel responsible for your cancer in any way?" The response I get can be quite angry, suggesting it is a cruel question. And yet if within themselves they feel it is cruel then it must in some way imply that there is a grain of truth which they do not wish to recognise. It is the dark side of the moon. I know how they feel. The question is cruel yet I feel that I can truly say "Yes, I am responsible for my cancer". Life at times to me is intolerable. I feel that the tasks imposed on me exceed my ability to perform; this is my weakness. My mental weakness. At times of this dis-ease within myself I feel a 'burn-out' mood descend. My whole body vitality is diminished, I am moody, sulky and very worried that my cancer is returning, increasing and so on. I know at times like this that I am impossible to live with; I feel it all over. Possibly it is a similar feeling to that experienced by women with PMT once a month. The hormone balance is upset and it is a temporary but natural upset. Now I hope I have learned to recognise these cancerous or pre-cancerous states of affair. Perhaps I will go quietly to the toilet and lock myself in and relax. "OK Colin, you cannot do anything just now, maybe it is not your place to do these outwardly self-imposed tasks within these self-imposed limits." I start to breath deeply and feel a change come over me as I cool down out of this tense state. I notice my hands sweating less. As my mental anxiety reduces my heart rate drops and I try within myself to bring myself to the state of mind that is right for me. The emotionally 'intolerable ' becomes 'tolerable' and allowing this change to continue upwards can bring matters to an 'achievable' state and even more. Achievers in life seem to have an instinct to be in the right place at the right time. The wind always seems to be in the right direction for them. They have instinctively learnt to rely on an inner way to guide them to their targets in life. They do not push along the same course if it is not producing the correct results. They alter their ways and attitudes to life and provided they keep that magic touch they (I feel) do not get cancer. Those who do get cancer are placing themselves under the kind of stress that is intolerable to their true self. Learn to recognise this in letting go. Go for a new way forward and know that it is right and proper for you. Do not try to blame; do not feel guilty; do not be imposed upon or try to impose tasks you cannot or do not wish to do; learn instead to re-draw the rules of life in your favour. This is a natural freedom to which we are all entitled.

Life is Love — For Enjoying

You might feel I am very serious person. All this natural food, healthy living, yoga and so on must be so boring! Life can't be worth living if such changes have to be made. If these are your views then I can assure you that you are wrong. I have made these changes and because of them *I am glad I had cancer!* It has been a lesson and certainly I am on a different path of life now. This path is excellent and you too can get on it as I keep encouraging you to do.

I now feel that I am doing the right things for myself. No longer am I a plodder in life. I am lucky in having a supportively loving wife and family who are great, but most of all I have a freedom that previously I did not possess. This freedom is entirely in the brain. It means I can enjoy life better by accepting the good things we all have and rejecting the bad things we don't require. So I take each day as it comes as I have earned it. I intend to savour the quality of that day to the full. I try totally to reject wallowing in thoughts of ghosts of the past, or anxiously awaiting the possible fates in store in the future. Can you follow what I am trying to convey to you? Possibly there is a confidence in myself that previously I lacked through worries both real and imagined. Those worries are now rejected and instead a feeling of warm love is within me. I still have some work to do on myself in this matter.

Some people try to find the feelings I now have by drinking, or in superficial relationships where the word 'love' is used when it should only be 'sex'. Superficial describes only those things which are outwardly apparent—skin deep rather than profoundly genuine or real. Through the work I have done on myself to come to terms with my cancer I find that I am avoiding the superficial instead of being attracted to it. You too must learn this lesson if you feel that up to now your life, relationships, etc have been on a shallow level. Consider your family and friends, for example, and decide whether they fit into one category rather than the other.

Relaxing with your cancer

The initial news of cancer brings with it a trek of well wishers and then a change takes place as the news sinks in and takes its full effect. Possibly the least expected people can suddenly be the most helpful and supportive to you. These people you encourage, and reward with thanks. Others, maybe even your nearest and dearest, seem to distance themselves and only call at dutiful intervals. Maybe they can't handle the problem; they have other matters on their minds; they have their own lives to lead. Just be prepared for this division and encourage those whom you find give you full support and accept you for what you are. To the rest just thank them kindly and if they cause distress ask them to wait until the time is right. You sort out the wheat from the chaff.

It follows that as you get better your friends who have helped you fall into a special love relationship which has been tempered in the furnace of cancer. Now you know your real friends and they receive that same profound gift from you. Arising from this excellence comes the new you, laughing and enjoying a totally new way of life. This is your aim and there is nothing to stop you finding this quality in your life but your own past negative life conditioning. So seek out this freedom, don't wait for it to happen as it will not happen *without your involvement*.

The Future

It would be nice to be optimistic about the future of cancer, that is to have some assurance that the numbers will drop and those who actually have cancer will have a greater chance of still surviving five years after the cancer manifests itself. A recent report made the prediction that by the year 2000 the five year survival rate for all cancers will increase to two persons out of three. This would mean a rate of say 60 to 70 per cent depending on whether you are male or female. The present 1987 figures are 30 per cent for men and 42 per cent for women. If this report proves correct then this will be good news. Let us look at some of the points it raises.

Lung cancer is the fourth largest killer disease; smoking is largely implicated here. The present trend of reducing smoking may make a significant contribution to improving the deaths overall in the future. My concern is the way we seem to allow the obvious to continue for many years without suitable action. Only recently has it been stated officially that smoking is a high risk factor in lung cancer. Even passive smoking puts a non-smoker at risk in a place where smoking is enjoyed by others. This information should have been made more widely known many years ago yet the excuse was that there was no actual proof. Now official health warnings are printed on cigarette packets. Why was this not done sooner—perhaps it might have saved a number of lives lost through lung cancer. To my regret I smoked until twenty years ago. I wish I had been more positively told about the real dangers I was placing my self into. I must blame my self for my stupidity.

Should we therefore look at other but similar dangers that surround us all? If my views on stress can be related to lung cancer via smoking, what else can we find? If we are capable of polluting the global self, then in similar ways we are capable of polluting our land, towns, cities, nations, the world. All of these pollution episodes can bring new problems, new stresses. My four-year-old medical reference book has no reference to AIDS. Is AIDS only the first of many new illnesses that are arising? Are all these problems of man's own making, as the results of smoking are to the individual?

We build new atomic power stations—the benefits of electricity are good. But what of the problems in the event of an accident? Radioactivity is dangerous; Japan still has a high incidence of cancer arising directly out of the two atomic bombs dropped in 1945. So forty years on the ghosts of the past invade the present—a typically cancerous situation. Atomic power stations do go wrong and can therefore cause higher rates of cancer. But for how long? How do the authorities dispose of the increase in nuclear waste? Send it out into the universe to extend pollution further and further? What happens when our power stations are decommissioned at the end of their useful life. Where does the radioactive waste go; how is it to be handled?

Then there is pollution by industry and individuals through the gases coming from exhausts. We have acid rain and acid air; at the same time we are destroying large tracts of the world's forests which enrich our atmosphere with the oxygen we need. What about land dusted by chemicals which leach into the soil and rivers to upset the cycle of life that existed before. Nitrates leach into our water supply—a fact that could be one of the causes of my stomach cancer. Who can say? Who can be sure? What about foods that are full of growth promoters, food and drink that leaves factories full of 'additives'? Maybe the products are more colourful, attractive, have a longer shelf life, are more profitable, but will they be more beneficial to us and give us what our bodies really need? I feel that each such product gives little at great cost and the body retains a little of those added chemicals which may build up into a toxic cocktail over which your defence systems have no control.

Then there are drugs such as the contraceptive pill or pain-killers which are prescribed in good faith by our doctors or which are bought carelessly over the counter and consumed in perhaps excessive quantities. We may have problems when these invading drugs actually fight against one another within our bodies: it is possible for instance for someone who takes the contraceptive pill to have its effect neutralised by a course of slimming pills and to become pregnant. If such a woman had not passed her rights of birth self control to others she would not be put in the position of having to give birth to an unwanted child. This is a particularly stressful problem—yet it is likely to become even commoner in the future unless collectively we take a different and more positive attitude to our self welfare.

The nature of balance

Every new venture or product brings good and bad; atomic power, the pill, asbestos—we have to weigh the balance and make our decisions from there. My house lies under the flight path from Heathrow Airport and we are constantly under strain because of the noise of passing jets. I would not try to grow vegetables in my garden as the exhausted air would diminish any food value. As it is we wash all our fruit and vegetables but we are never sure that it is all wholesome. What about our water supply? You can see now why the matter of purification is essential. We may have made advances in hygiene but to what extent are the advantages offset in other areas, adding to the sum total of all our stresses? Many feel as I do and what I write may be understood by you. Possibly you can see that in the same way as toxins and other stresses can build up in the body to overwhelm the defence systems so too can the world about you be affected in a similar manner. These enemies are unseen and unfelt until sufficient in numbers to create new cancerous situations.

That is why I feel so passionately that you, dear friend, are aware of all the causes of your cancer and that you do something to help yourself. I am not alone in my views, in fact if it hadn't been for many others guiding and advising me, then I would not be alive and in such good health today. Remember though: it was up to me to accept or reject as I decided and that is what I trust you have been learning to do. So my dear friend what are you going to do for the future? What have you already done since starting to read this book? Your diary should give you the answer and show the progress you have made. I hope so. Are you now healthier, wiser, more confident, more understanding, more tolerant and more loving? I trust you will continue along the path I have been guiding you along up to now.

Continuing your quest

In the final Chapter I list the organisations, books, audio tapes, etc that have been helpful to me in some way and may be helpful to you. This book is after all only a stepping stone in your fight and you must never give up that fight. You will still be in need of extra help *after* reading this book. It is after all written from a patient's point of view and then only with the knowledge that has been acquired in a relatively short space of time. The actual presence of qualified people, a medical advisor, a cancer counsellor, is worth much more than a book such as this. As an example of what I mean let me add that we are all unique and some of us instantly follow what another advises. Alternatively, I know that many people would not comprehend any aspect of spiritual growth and would close up their minds totally. In counselling such people it would obviously be unhelpful to speak about such matters as this would destroy the close relationship of confidence that has to be built. Slowly and surely the counsellor enlarges the area of discussion until the subject comes into the conversation almost naturally. In a one-to-one discussion the patient does all the talking—well most of it—whereas here I have had to do all the writing. I have written blind if you like, because I know nothing about you and you know a great deal about me.

A special message

Remember everything that I have written that has special importance to you. (Remember that suggestion given at the beginning of the book, to mark passages that have meaning for you, and to make notes in the margin). I have given of my best for your good. I was helped by a great team who pushed me forward and pulled me upwards when I needed it. So let us all push and pull together into the future—with happiness, with love.

Chapter 12

COMMUNICATIONS

Passing the Message on to Your Spouse, Companion or Carer

This final Chapter is not so much for the cancer patient as for the cancer patient's spouse, close companion or carer. Their needs are just as important. They need to know your inner feelings, your inner fears, your panics, your loneliness, your concern over the future. They need to understand that in some way the past relationship is being tested and tried and that 'the cancer' is able to grow between you as an insidious enemy that may cut the bonds of your love between each other. This must not happen and you must be in harmony with the other. My aim in this Chapter is to help the spouse or carer understand deeply your innermost problems and to recognise that rather than allow the cancer problem to drive you apart, it should serve to draw you together.

This drawing together is a reaffirmation of your love for each other which can suddenly and wonderfully improve your relationship so that each of you finds hidden qualities and weaknesses which you share. It is joyful. Suddenly this bond between you takes on a whole new meaning and the quality of your lives is improved beyond measure. It is as if in battle you are finding the true meaning of the expression comrade in arms, chum, pal, friend, lover, or whatever in your relationship you are to each other. Sharing troubles reduces the pain so learn to open out one to another in total awareness that now you really need your love for each other.

A list of organisations and books that are helpful to cancer patients is given at the end of the letter that follows. You will find that there are plenty of others but I hope that you will find the help you need—or a start to the help you need—from the ones I have included.

Colin

A Letter to the Spouse or Carer

Dear Friend,

So you are caring for a cancer patient.

Well, you have a problem, haven't you? You probably feel unfit to handle it. You may feel that this matter is the responsibility of the doctors. It is up to them to produce a cure and then you can all go on as before.

Can you take that chance? Can you just sit down and do nothing at all to assist? Is it alright to be able to make just a few remarks intended to be helpful? "How long do you reckon?" "What does the doctor suggest to you?"

NO YOU CAN'T! SORRY . . . NO! NO! NO!

Cancer is a dangerous disease. It is not just a growth that can spread in the body. It is a disease of the whole person. Cancer can only exist in a body when that body has been brought down to such a bad state that the defence system has collapsed. This defence immune system is governed by the mind and passes to all parts of the body. So the mind is not doing its protective job either.

However, cancer can go further by causing a parting in your relationship by coming between you and the one you love or care for. Surely you cannot allow this to happen. Good! So you're going to be in there helping in every way possible. Yes? OK!

You must remove all the barriers that exist in your relation-ship to each other. In many ways you will need to forget your pride and to do things you never ever thought possible. Suddenly you have to pitch in together and become a pair of people who together fight the cancer on all levels.

Removing the barriers is the first hurdle between you and your patient. The doctor has a desk between the patient and himself. That barrier will always exist however good a friend the doctor is. The doctor needs to protect himself from becoming excessively involved in any one patient. He has other patients as well and he needs to protect himself in a professional manner in the matter of any doctor/patient relationship.

You have the advantage here—you can be the active force that allows any such barrier to be removed. You may not fully understand what I am trying to say so I will give an example of a wife with cancer whom I went to see. We talked together for some hours with her husband present. Suddenly the husband said that he could see what I was trying to find in their relationship. "Colin, in this house, we live as if we are guests in a guest house. We each have our own separate beds, chairs, interests. We don't touch each other and even our meals are different". The wife cried and I felt that when I left their house it had become their home (rather than a guest house) and the barriers slowly erected over the years of their relationship had fallen away. This was the beginning of a new way forward.

Grief is a marvellous way to upset the barriers that exist in a relationship and it is totally correct for you to grieve either with your patient or alone if you so wish. Learning to grieve together is good as it releases stress and you have as much right to weep as your patient. It shows that you too have needs of your own space and that you have love for the cancer victim.

Space to talk to each other is very important. Turn off the television set and deal with other possible distractions; allow each of you to talk to the other without any interruption. Find out if anything has gone wrong with your love for each other. Have you both been totally truthful! Do you need to confess some past mistake or mistakes to each other. Learn to do it. Probably the other knows the truth anyway and it just needs to be said out loud to remove that weed from your garden of love for each other.

Give permission to each other to confess, to say you are sorry one to the other, to repay debts however owed, and then, joy of joy, to forgive the other. What a release! Forgive them for they know not what they do. An example of this was a husband who asked to see me alone in his home. Hour after hour went by as he took me through his cancer history. The story started when he first felt a pain but I knew that was not the start. That was only the manifestation of the cancer. The start was much earlier than that but you can't rush these things. Finally, after he had talked himself dry I said "What do you hold within you that you haven't said?" This was I felt a dangerous question as I might have to listen to his cancer story all over again from the manifestation! However, he suddenly burst out that a few weeks before the cancer was discovered he had been caught stealing. He tried to hide his crime from his family; he had no need to steal and so on. He was ashamed. He could not see that he was punishing himself and he could not bring himself to the point of telling his family. Finally I persuaded him to go to the toilet and indicated that during his absence I would reveal his problem. Thankfully, after some initial misgivings, he agreed to this.

When his wife and son came in I asked them to sit down and implied that I had unearthed a problem that might be the cause of the cancer, "It might not be the only cause but at least it is a start." "Please tell us Colin. Anything we can do to help him and keep the family happy and together will be wonderful." "Your husband's cancer is driving you apart from him because he has been stupid and he is punishing himself. Just forgive and I am sure things will start going better for all of you from now on." I explained his misdeed, how upset he was over it and how he was punishing himself so that his self respect had gone.

"Is that all it is", said his wife. "Of course I forgive him. I can't allow such a thing to stand between us and cause all this anxiety; it is so stupid, so trivial". She repeated this to her husband when he returned and they both burst into tears in each other's arms. Even his son had I felt grown in strength by knowing that parents, like children, have weaknesses as well as strengths. Forgiving—to ask for it and to receive it—is an essential lubricating oil of love.

Strangely, finding out the emotional causes of cancer will provide strength in renewed bonds of love; all at once the way forward seems clear as an important barrier has been overcome. I have found that cancer has given me a new freedom that previously I did not have. I have used the knowledge within my self that when you come so close to death then there is nothing to fear from life. This does not mean breaking laws but it does mean breaking codes and conventions we have been conditioned to accept during our growing up.

Learning to listen more carefully to other views and beliefs is part of the growth we all need in our lives. Some of the information I retain, some is discarded as not being for me just at the moment. This is part of one's journey through life. Before if you like my life was in a rut leading to a grave, now it is not. Frankly it is all a mental attitude within ourselves which has to atune to those who live and work with us. It is a constantly changing pattern of pressures on your self which goes on all the time. You need to understand how the cancer can divide you and your loved one (s) as a team and keep you apart in the same way as it can divide body cells. Your direction in loving care is to become more united than before. See if this works for you.

Cancer — a definition

A malignant growth or tumour of any type caused by uncontrolled and abnormal division of the body cells. It is an evil growth that can spread its corrupting canker through the host body.

Cancer — the opposite

A lovingly enriched normal body in which the body cells function correctly in the way nature intended. The cells have a birth, life and a replacement to continue the rhythm of the host body's life cycle.

This freedom from past social conditioning is what we all need to grasp, you as well as your patient. Just unlock those mental shackles and together step out into a new life. There is probably no reason why you can't both go on the holiday of a lifetime to fulfil that desire of a lifetime that you both have. To see and hear the opera in Milan, to fly a kite, paint in the Lake District, hang glide, bobsleigh down the Cresta, see the grandchildren in New Zealand—whatever is your dream fulfillment. Why not?

Perhaps you will discover that you are cutting the old bonds that have repressed you so that they have grown like nooses around your neck; even a family can leach you dry with their daily demands. Until I had cancer I had never ridden a motor-cycle. Now I find a freedom in doing just that. I use that joy in a practical way in riding to and from work. I transfer the boring commuter train journey into an adventure which I admit—having just been knocked off my bike—is not without its dangers. However, even that negative incident, my motorcycle accident, has proved positive to me in allowing me to finish writing this book.

Following my accident I noticed that the healing of my injured leg was slow because of the chemotherapy treatment that I had been having for my cancer. This reminds me to point out how important it is that your patient washes properly and is clean at all times. Any cut, however small, must be treated properly. Hair and nails must be cut short because cancer treatments upset the body's healing functions. Try to ensure that your patient wears clothes made from natural (but brightly coloured) materials and that the food you both eat is natural and eaten slowly in prayer if that is your desire. Yes, I did write 'both'! If you are to help your patient then you must be wholly involved (in body, mind and spirit) in all treatments other than the medical ones. This means that you eat the same food and enjoy it together. You have healing, meditate, do yoga and so on together. It is no good taking your patient to some treatment and saying you would rather stay outside or go for a smoke. You are needed: to help, advise and speak out when the patient is too fearful and tongue-tied. This means total togetherness so that you can in all honesty say "We had cancer and survived".

Remember you yourself might be the cause of the cancer. You

145

can easily annoy your patient by your funny little ways and by habits which upset. You may need the holistic treatments you agree upon just as much as your patient. You can't treat just a half, you have to treat the whole, holistically. Each person lives by *prana* which is the energy life force. When you are alive it governs your every moment like electricity giving light to a lamp. Turn it off by reducing the power and nothing is the result. The light from that bulb continues into space for infinity but the source is dead. Your patient needs to have a plentiful source of power and this they get from good food, drink, the air they breathe and the other life forces that surround us. Your love is ensuring that the power is provided in full measure.

When I was very ill I existed solely on grapes and mild herbal teas. Soon this diet expanded to include other simple natural foods and wholemeal bread. I ate little and often so as to keep my body functioning and fighting. Rosemary, my wife, helped me with this diet. Cancer is a battle and you must, for your own good, understand how important it is to win it. Do not just allow despair to sweep over you both. This approach means a total commitment and no half measures.

"But what do I do Colin?"

Strangely, the answer is almost nothing. You both learn to meditate twice a day together. Yes it is difficult, but it is not impossible. Our lives are so full of noise, clutter and high energy levels that to sit comfortably, quietly for two twenty-minute periods, once in the morning and once in the evening is not easy. Yet it must be done. Just agree that there are to be no interruptions. This is a time of soul space. You are both souls seeking and receiving. You need to communicate silently not only with each other but also with a source which is there but not often heard. Just listen and you will know what to do.

Writing this book was the last thing I ever considered and yet I was encouraged to do so when the publishers heard through one of their employees of my cancer. A communication came through. Frankly my first feelings on being asked to write this book were: No! An ego trip! What have I got to say that hasn't been better said, better researched in every way, is better value— and anyway are there not enough books on cancer already?

Rosemary reminded me that just suppose that one person,

somewhere, sometime, decided to take some life saving action as a result of reading a few words from this book, perhaps words uttered to me by others now dead. Can I possibly allow a break to occur in that chain of the message, whatever it may be? This book has driven me to tears, to deep desperation. I have had to give of my inner feelings for you and for your patient. You could be my family in name but we are all family and wholly inter-related, helping and receiving from each other. Can you deny your knowledge to others? In my meditation I learn to listen, not with my ears but by an intuitive inner mental receiver. Once that is happening my awareness is opened and messages start flooding into my mind. It is as if, as I have explained earlier in the book, I were a deep pond. The mud on the bottom generates a tiny bubble of thought which flows upwards to the surface, expanding and joining with others. In our life we call this a 'good idea'. You need lots of those!

Meditation requires discipline to do it and your obedient acceptance of what is given and received. What you discover may be difficult and a challenge, but do it and don't be put off by what seems to be impossible. Learn to have the freedom to explore new areas and to share those experiences with others. In this way things start going your way together. Never discuss your worries behind your patient's back, however well meaning. Learn to talk of death easily and if it comes then the one left behind has the freedom of a new life and not the shackles of bereavement. Totally draw the family into your plans when the decisions have been made as they have every right to know and will feel hurt if you leave them out.

Understand and respect the wishes of your patient who may have family and friends they do not really love or wish to see. Simply talk it through together. Do not act separately in this matter as you will lose all trust and cancer will be the victor. Realise that a relationship has different values. One partner may rely more on the other and this creates an imbalance and is wrong. A team works equally together in balanced harmony so permit an adjustment to be made so that you are in tune. Allow your home to be filled with music you love and flowers that give a message of peace. This new spirit of enhanced love will encourage people to come to visit you both rather than to be frightened away by fear. Do not allow cancer to dominate your lives in any way, shape or form. Treat it with the contempt it deserves and act appropriately. Cancer is an invader; kick it out! Remember that the five-year diary must be completed on a regular basis. You have a five-year plan for joint cancer survival and it can be a cornerstone in your lives. What interesting reading it will make.

A sexual relationship if you have one is vital. Do not be put off by all that is said or implied about it. If you are actually considering a pregnancy then it would be wise to get medical advice first as chemotherapy can have bad effects on the unborn child. There is however no need to deny each other the comfort and need of courtship leading up to sex even if the sex fulfillment is for the time being unobtainable. A hand lovingly slipped under the blanket can remind each other of the good things in life to be enjoyed in the future. If you have a good sense of humour then allow this area of your lives to be opened up in a loving way. "Does that drip contraption mean that you will be more virile in the future?" "Can you be trusted with all those pretty nurses/handsome doctors around?"

Ideally the patient needs to spend only the shortest time in hospital and will improve best in a loving home atmosphere. It is a help when your patient is in hospital if they can dress in something clean, colourful and cheerful. Colour is very important and can mean a lot to the overall improvement and well-being of your patient. A track suit in some natural material is better than bed wear and dressing gown. Somehow a patient looks more well and certainly feels better in themselves.

Rosemary always brings a touch of humour and love into my life. Without her I can feel quite despondent. I realise just how hard she has worked in my survival. Together we have made it, together, with the help of others. Nevertheless we are ordinary people, unique, just like everybody else. We are however prepared to do whilst others perhaps might just talk and discuss. Sometimes what we do is wrong in hindsight, but we did it and we learnt our lesson and that is what is important. Learn to do. We like to feel that we generate a ring or light of confidence to those we see with cancer. This ring or light is easy to acquire. You just know that what you both decide to do is right then you go ahead and do it together. Surely you have experienced that feeling that nothing could go wrong, and nothing did. This is confidence or good morale and if troops are instilled with such confidence then battles are won against impossible odds. Battles are lost by lack of morale. There is no spirit in defeat, only dispiritment.

Cancer is a kind of 'fifth column' enemy in your patient's body and small though it may be it can spread rapidly if conditions are suitable for growth. Your aim is to help your patient to reverse the whole negativity of their body, improve their defences and survive.

This book is only a step in your life together. Care well for your patient as well as yourself. Learn the lessons together.

Colin

Organisations (1995 Update)

When I was asked to bring the first edition of this book up to date it was interesting to see that most of the organisations originally listed had moved from their old addresses. In six years a lot of change takes place. There is nothing more despairing than to be given a list of organisations to contact and find that it is of little use. So this time I have reduced the list to five charities. They should be able to help you get started forming your network of local help. The first stage is to learn where the local cancer support groups are and from them you will discover whatever is available that is suitable for you.

There is much to be done, so it is a question of getting your doctor, nurses, supportive family and friends organised as your personal team. Between them they can find out what is needed to get a network of assistance, it will be just a telephone call away. Team spirit is the key and all their findings will be recorded into your five year diary. This indicates a practical commonsense orderly state of mind. Part of the healing process is seeking help constantly. The desire to discover what is right for you starts the transformational process away from the "old" to the "new" you. That is exactly what has happened to me and contributed to my health.

Your team will search out a wide range of local assistance offering "Holistic, Alternative, Complementary or Natural Medicine". Once you find what is right then health improvement evolves. Change starts slowly and surely day by day, similar to the transformation from chrysalis into butterfly, or buds into flowers. Ideally the healing techniques used will harmonize with all the natural requirements and rhythms of the person taking the process of well-being well beyond the scope of conventional medicine.

1. Bristol Cancer Help Centre
(Registered Charity No. 284881)
Grove House, Cornwallis Grove, Clifton, Bristol, Avon, BS8 4PG
Tel. Bristol (01272) 743216.
Weekly residential and non-residential holistic courses for cancer patients which include counselling, relaxation, visualisation, meditation, art therapy, healing, dietary advice and vitamin supplements. Provides seminars and workshops for general and specialist groups and an education programme.

2. BACUP
(Registered Charity No. 290526)
3 Bath Place, Rivington Street, London EC2A 3JR
Freephone: (0800) 181199 Mon-Thu 10-7, Fri 10-5.30.
London callers: (0171) 613 2121. Counselling: (0171) 696 9000.
Cancer nurses provide information and emotional support to patients, relatives and friends. London based one-to-one counselling services which are free.

3. CancerLink
(Registered Charity No. 326430)
17 Britannia Street, London WC1X 9JN
Tel. Information Service: (0171) 833 2451. 9.30-5.30.
Self Help & Support Service: (0171) 833 2818. 9.30-5.30.
Provide emotional support and information about all aspects of cancer. Assistance and training to cancer self help and support groups, help set up new groups. Offers advice to young people and ethnic minorities.

4. British Wheel of Yoga
(Registered Charity No. 264993)
1 Hamilton Place, Boston Road, Sleaford, Lincs. NG34 7ES
Tel: (01529) 306851.
This charity will provide full information on qualified yoga teachers through a network of Regional and County representatives throughout the United Kingdom. They have connections with yoga organisations elsewhere in the world.

5. The Association for New Approaches to Cancer
(Registered Charity No. 285530)
5 Larksfield, Englefield Green, Egham, Surrey TW20 0RB
Tel. (01784) 433610.
The Association was conceived in 1969 and received its charitable status in 1982. This Charity promotes the benefits of complementary, holistic and self-help methods of healing. Slowly, conventional medical hospitals are opening up and becoming aware of these new approaches to cancer as patients and enlightened persons seek extra help.

The Charity acts as a nerve centre for a network of local cancer self-help groups, complementary and holistic practitioners, therapists, clinics, yoga classes, recommended books, nutritional guide-lines and so on throughout the United Kingdom and overseas.

The Charity provides a unique service for each person's needs. This depends on what is required, on where that person is in their treatment. All methods of Healing, Therapies and Natural medicine are collected, nothing is rejected.

I work as the Honorary Secretary and our home has become the office of the Charity. Our team of workers are spread in this country and abroad all inspired to help and some with past cancer experience. My wife, Rosemary, has this message stuck on her desk:

"We are all spiritual beings coping with human life ...
not humans trying to be spiritual."

When writing to these organisations enclose a LARGE stamped addressed envelope. A small envelope expects a short reply?

To Sum Up

There is so much I am learning and wish to share with you. I know there is only so much anyone can absorb. Have faith in the miracles of new life as you transform yourself.

Do not live in the fear of despair, that makes matters worse. I know that feeling of being alone in the middle of a busy world, of thinking that nobody has the time for you anymore.

Know that there are hands that heal, ears that listen, arms which enfold, shoulders to share that load, and hearts overflowing with love. Just know that the more you search, the more you secure. The mind tensions of fear can be gathered up tight, spun around and drawn out into ropes of strength, confidence and belief.

Read how an American sums up this book. You know it is an American by the spelling!

"Cancer isn't a growth that can spread in your body: it is a disease of the whole person. Cancer can only exist in a body whose natural immune system has reached a weakened state. These defenses of the immune system are controlled by the mind and pass to all parts of the body, so when the mind reaches a weakened state, it allows the body to become susceptible to cancer.

'Following his own bout with cancer, author Colin Ryder Richardson has written a warm and sensitive book describing his personal experiences. His book, "Mind Over Cancer", provides comfort and counsel as well as a wealth of information about the dis-ease and the sort of stresses that can foster it. Colin leads the reader through the research he did to help himself through his own illness, and on the way, reflects on the past, and more importantly, discusses what can be done for the present. Touching on topics from diet and exercise to yoga and prayer, from relaxation techniques to affirmations like humour and "letting go", to visualizing and strengthening your will to live, the author explains the important role played by the mind in arresting the dis-ease."

Cancer is a very complex dis-ease. The unique workings of our minds and attitudes we adopt are just as complex. Ask anybody how the mind works and you will get different answers.

Imagine you are an observer. Ask yourself two questions:
1. Positive attitude, "Has my body always enjoyed clear cut directions from my calm mind?" (Ease).
and then:
2. Negative attitude: "Has my mind been in continual conflict over my past problems, present confusions and future uncertainties, sending out erratic, contradictory, timid, nervous messages? Causing my pulse to race? ALL of which lets my body suffer?" (Dis-ease).

Which answer more truly applies to you? Naturally we must work towards the positive attitude.

Recently I bought a book "Introduction to Psychology". It was first published in 1953 and is now in its fortieth year. The book has over 800 pages and claims to be the most popular current standard reference book for students. In the chapter "Stress and Coping" it includes "New" sections on how stress affects health. (Notice the word "New"!) The medical profession now gives names:
Psychoimmunology! and Psychoneuroimmunology!
or for short ("PI" and "PNI").
1. "PI" is the study of how the body's immune system is affected by Stress or similar factors.
2. "PNI" is the study of the mind's ability to affect change in the body.

Basically if you accept that "PI" has allowed cancer to manifest within, then there is a need to adopt "PNI" to resolve it.

Here is a simple form of questionnaire:
Negative answers are in brackets as examples given to me by those who do not wish to make a change, that is their freedom of choice.
1. Honestly examine your life in detail. Have you trod a wrong path so that you have cancer? What are the causes? List in your five year diary those negative things which have upset you. Reject or resolve them ruthlessly. This includes "Deep Inner Fears" which I mentioned at the start. Are you prepared to do this?

(Yes Colin but . . . so much seems to have gone wrong in my life. In the past few years, ever since . . . died/divorced/went away/lonely etc . . .).

153

2. Know you are the most important person in your life and until you are in good health (Mind, Body and Spirit), you cannot attend or even think of attending to the problems of others. This is a selfish attitude which you need to adopt. Can you do that and let go? A person with cancer caused by stress will find this hard. Their attitude is unselfish care for others, excessive devotion to family, work and so on, and little or no concern for themselves.

(Yes Colin, but . . . I never seem to have time for myself, I seem to be so busy looking after . . .").

So who gets hurt?

3. Do you feel needed? Loved unconditionally? Listened to? Supported?

("Yes Colin, but . . . all that love you talk about went and does not now exist in my life. I am lonely, others have moved on . . . Children have left home").

4. Do you feel self confident? Have you the will and single determination to seek health through change? Attitude? Diet? Friends? Music? Colour? Laughter? a change of direction, etc?

("Yes Colin, but . . . I just feel so tired these days. I just can't . . .").

5. Is there a deep meaning within your life? Do you feel secure with that? Have you things to do for yourself? Ambitions? Holidays?

("Yes Colin, but . . . those things I had and did but not now. I can't think about anything anymore . . .").

6. Do you feel a sense of profound fulfilment and contentment, are you truly happy?

(No Colin! . . . to be honest, life now seems so hard, so sad. I don't remember when I last had fun or a laugh.").

7. Do you have a constant passionate desire to make wholesome changes to the way you: Live (I just exist), Think (I worry), Eat (Junk Food), Exercise (Lack of Body Activity), Sleep (Lie Awake), Relationships and Work (Unsatisfactory), and Everything else you do even down to the type and colour of clothes you wear?

("Look Colin, there seems so much . . .").

8. Are you open minded, prepared to accept personal responsibility for your thoughts, actions and health?

("Now Colin, I see it this way, I leave everything to the doctors and do exactly what they say. Nothing else. They are the experts, what's the point ...").

9. Do you understand the hoilistic approach of Body, Mind and Spirit? and how they connect?

(Well Colin, I do and I might try hard but my husband ...").

10. Do you have a quiet mind that is free, without distresses such as fear, worry, jealousy, anger, envy? Do you suppress these negative emotions when they erupt?

(Please Colin, I keep myself to myself. Yes I admit I do fret if everything is not right. Yes, I do keep my temper, bite my tongue, well that is right isn't it? They call that being stoic, don't they?").

11. Can you forgive others and ask for forgiveness? Can you accept changes?

("Oh! Colin. How can I ever forgive after all that happened ...? I have never spoken about this before, it started ... Why should I?").

12. Will you be prepared to discipline your life exclusively to your personal well-being and let those who love you care for you, rather than you for them?

(No Colin, I cannot forget my obligations, I cannot change. I have always ... Can I get you a cup of tea? biscuit? cake? or something? surely you need something don't you? having come all that way ... ?").

If you recognise yourself with those negative answers, then you know now how to readdress your attitudes. Readers' reactions to the first edition of this book have been wholly supportive, encouraging and stimulating. If I have inspired them to get well then it is only because I have been equally encouraged by others. Inspiration is the breathe of Spirit and that is how it inspires.

I have met people who go round with this book in their hands, faithfully marking it with notes in the margins as I have suggested, writing their own dedications on the inside covers, composing poems of love and beautiful messages to other readers, and that includes books on loan from the local library! There seems to be groups endorsing borrowed copies with a desire to share lifeline messages with each other. (Healthy people will not understand this but do not let their ignorance put you off.) It is a humbling and enlightening experience to meet people who are definitely changing for a better way. You can tell that from their excitement and light in their eyes. It is like the sun suddenly coming out on a dull day so that everything glows warmly into all the colours of the spectrum. Understand that this profound alteration within is natural healing at work. You have everything to gain and enjoy, just like falling in love.

The challenge and message of this book is the knowledge that cancer clearly points to a basic truth that mental confusion festers the body. Let this book alter your whole being with a great surge of healing energy, if it works for me than it will work for you!

Finally I offer you advice from the WHICH magazine, "WHICH? WAY TO HEALTH". They confirm that common-sense suggests taking the best of both worlds, namely combining the benefits of modern drugs and high technology with the more holistic care that is offered by Bristol Cancer Help Centre, New Approaches to Cancer and the like.

Why not write to me care of the publishers:
W. Foulsham & Co. Ltd.
(Department CRR)
The Publishing House
Bennetts Close, Cippenham, Berkshire SL1 5AP
or direct to me at:
New Approaches to Cancer, enclosing a large stamped addressed envelope. The address was provided earlier under "Organisations". Tell me about yourself. Are you able to identify to the twelve questions? How can I help you further and can you help this Charity?

Love,
WHAT IS LIFE? = Love, Inspiration, Faith, Energy.
Faith,
Energy.

Colin

Books to Read

The Bible

Getting Well Again, O Carl Simonton, MD, Stephanie Matthews-Simonton, James L Creighton, Bantam Books, 1980
This book is excellent. It describes the typical 'cancer personality' and aspects of stress and other emotional factors. It explains meditation techniques such as visualisation so that your self help and self care can be an important weapon in the war on cancer. I have listened to both Carl and Stephanie talk and found them very understanding.

You Can Conquer Cancer, Ian Gawler, Thorsons, 1986
Another excellent book. Ian is a vet so he has medical knowledge yet he writes at a level of understanding that is easy to follow about his own cancer experiences. There is much helpful information on diet and many other aspects I mention in the main body of the book.

Opening Doors Within, Eileen Caddy, The Findhorn Press, The Park, Forres IV36 OTZ, Scotland, 1986
Eileen is a co-founder of the Findhorn Foundation in Scotland. Send for the catalogue but I recommend that you order the above book especially. The book gives an inspirational message for each day of the year and makes a lovely present to someone you love—which of course includes yourself.

Champion's Story, Bob Champion and Jonathan Powell, Fontana, 1981

Understanding Cancer, Consumer's Association, publishers of Which?, 1986
This is a factual book and helpful in explaining what your doctor may omit to mention or expand on.

The Cancer Reference Book, Paul M Levitt and Elissa S Guralnick with Dr A Robert Kagan and Dr Harvey Gilbert, Paddington Press, 1979

Good-bye to Guilt, Gerald G Jampolsky MD, Bantam Books, 1985
You should be able to get this book from the Centre for Attitudinal Healing, PO Box 638, London SW3 4LN. Other books by the same author: *Love is Letting Go of Fear* and *Teach Only Love*

The Topic of Cancer, Dick Richards, Pergamon Press, 1982

You Can Fight For Your Life, Lawrence LeShan, Thorsons, 1984
This is a really good book. All cancer patients should read it and the others written by Lawrence such as *Holistic Health* and *How to Meditate*. The author is also a first class speaker

The Wealth Within, Ainslie Meares MD, Ashgrove Press, 1984
Ainslie is a lovely man and writes well.

Does Diet Cure Cancer, Dr Maud Tresillian Fere, Thorsons, 1971

Now That You Have Cancer, Robert W Bradford, Choice Publications, Los Altos, Ca, USA, 1977

On Death and Dying, Elisabeth Kübler-Ross, MD, Tavistock Publications, 1973

On Children and Death, Elisabeth Kübler-Ross, MD, Macmillan Publishing, New York, 1983

Living With Death and Dying, Elisabeth Kübler-Ross, Souvenir Press, 1982
I enjoyed a week's course with Elisabeth and found her methods of caring for those in a terminal situation to be profoundly loving. Elisabeth is a spirited fighter for those in need during the period of dying and afterwards during the period of bereavement.

Freedom from Stress, Alethea Lawson, Thorsons, 1978

The Whole Health Manual, Patrick Holford, Thorsons, 1983

Vitamin Vitality, Patrick Holford, Collins, 1985

New Approaches to Cancer, Shirley Harrison, Century, 1987

Why Meditation, Swami Shyam, A Be All Publication, 1983

The Sovereign Secret of Meditation, Swami Shyam, published by Pierre Schenk (for Shyam's Institute of Higher Knowledge), 1974

Angela's Bookshop
65 Norfolk Road
Seven Kings
Ilford, Essex
IG3 8LJ
(01 599 0865)
This shop is run by Angela and Ken Thompson. It has a good range of yoga books and music and relaxation tapes. To enter into the right mood to meditate, it is helpful to play quiet music to change the brain wave patterns to a more subdued level. Angela and Ken are both excellent yoga teachers as well as being our good friends.

These are only a few of the organisations and books that have helped me on my way. Some of the information I have disregarded as not being for me; other points have been literally life saving. You in turn must not limit yourself to looking for just 'one cure'; 'one method'. Your approach must take account of many factors including age, the extent and location of the cancer, and the true desire to get better. 'My' approach was right for me, I now know where I went wrong in my life. It all began many years ago and bit by bit I slipped downhill, however hard I tried to climb back up again. Cancer was the turning point and I found I had to change my direction and my attitudes. Two years before I even thought of writing this book I was visited by Ralph Barker who at that time was researching his book called *Children of the Benares* (published by Methuen in 1987). I haven't yet read the finished book but if you want to learn more about the incident I mention on pages 21 and 120, the one that relates to the initial cause of my cancer, I recommend that you read it.

May 1987, Surrey